Praise for *THE DEATH OF CANCER*

"For the past half century, [DeVita] has been at the forefront of the fight against one of the world's most feared diseases, and in *The Death of Cancer* he has written an extraordinary chronicle . . . His conclusions are deeply unsettling . . . DeVita's portrait of the way things were gives us a glimpse of what the future may look like."

—Malcolm Gladwell, *The New Yorker*

"A surprising and riveting story." —Jenni Laidman, *Chicago Tribune*

"In *The Death of Cancer*, Dr. DeVita (with his daughter Elizabeth DeVita-Raeburn) paints a portrait of a cancer industrial complex desperately in need of an overhaul, hampered by petty politics and power mongering, among much else . . . Powerful . . . There is no mistaking the value of the core idea he wants to convey: that doctors and researchers commit themselves anew to doing everything possible to help the patient." —Laura Landro, *The Wall Street Journal*

"An authoritative review of the history of surgery and radiation therapy . . . Ultimately, DeVita ably shows that the development of oncology as a modern specialty is a very human story."

—Sandeep Jauhar, *The New York Times Book Review*

"This riveting, beautifully written, and poignant memoir takes us on an enormous journey—from cancer's past to its future. Vincent T. DeVita Jr. brings us behind the scenes to the invention of breakthrough therapies for some forms of cancer in the 1960s and '70s. He also provides a much-needed manifesto for the future."

—Siddhartha Mukherjee, Pulitzer Prize–winning author of *The Emperor of All Maladies*

"An utterly absorbing memoir, fierce and frank . . . The average reader will come away from the book with a superb basic education in all things oncological, from events on the cellular level to those in the rooms where research agendas are settled and checks are written."

—Abigail Zuger, M.D., *The New York Times*

"If ever a book about cancer could offer hope for the future, it's this one." —Joselin Linder, *New York Post*

"Dr. Vincent DeVita is an eminent oncologist . . . [who] became adept not only in cancer medicine but in cancer politics . . . DeVita rightly argues [that] we are now at a much better place than we were in past decades." —Jerome Groopman, *The New York Review of Books*

"Fascinating . . . Siddhartha Mukherjee called his Pulitzer Prize–winning *The Emperor of All Maladies* a 'biography' of the disease. *The Death of Cancer* is its obituary. We're at 'the beginning of the end,' DeVita declares of the war on cancer."

—Suzanne Koven, *The Boston Globe*

"In this engaging, provocative, and deeply personal book, Vincent DeVita and Elizabeth DeVita-Raeburn provide a compelling insider's guide into the personalities, organizations, and key protagonists that provided the backdrop and impetus for this unprecedented campaign . . . *The Death of Cancer* presents a candid and disarming critique of the ways in which medicine, and specifically oncology, is regulated in the United States." —Adrian Woolfson, *Science*

"Great scientists are not always great writers, but this book is a welcome exception, being well-crafted, compelling, transparent, and overall, optimistic." —Jules Morgan, *The Lancet Oncology*

"An extraordinary book and an extraordinary story."

—Otis W. Brawley, *The Cancer Letter*

"[A] straight-talking, optimistic memoir." —Tony Miksanek, *Booklist*

"Superb science writing . . . One of the most absorbing and empowering science histories to hit the shelves in recent years."
—*Kirkus Reviews* (starred review)

"DeVita blends crisp writing and a gift for explaining complicated scientific concepts clearly with deep knowledge, passion, and wit. The book is by turns entertaining and maddening but always fascinating. Highly recommended." —Janet Crum, *Library Journal* (starred review)

"DeVita, an oncologist and professor at Yale School of Medicine, collaborates with his daughter DeVita-Raeburn on this engaging, informative, and inspiring history of DeVita's prominent role in developing innovative cancer treatments . . . This remarkable memoir doesn't just urge the public to have hope: it showcases the exciting evidence that we may finally be winning the war on cancer."
—*Publishers Weekly* (starred review)

"*The Death of Cancer* is an astonishingly good read. Written by a cancer expert who happens to be a cancer survivor as well, it deftly explains the treatments that have turned this insidious disease from a death sentence into a manageable chronic condition for millions of people—and what yet remains to be done. I devoured the book in two sittings, struck, page after page, by its insight, honesty, compassion, and plain common sense." —David M. Oshinsky, Pulitzer Prize–winning author of *Polio: An American Story*

"*The Death of Cancer* is a fascinating insider history of the long battle against one of the world's most feared diseases, told with both insight and frustration, and ultimately with hope. This collaboration between the former National Cancer Institute director Vincent T. DeVita Jr. and his talented science writer daughter, Elizabeth DeVita-Raeburn, results in a wonderfully human portrait of the scientists who join the fight and a wonderfully smart look at the ways we might actually win it."
—Deborah Blum, *New York Times* bestselling author of *The Poisoner's Handbook*

ALSO BY VINCENT T. DeVITA JR., M.D.

DeVita, Hellman, and Rosenberg's Cancer:
Principles & Practice of Oncology

ALSO BY ELIZABETH DeVITA-RAEBURN

The Empty Room:
Understanding Sibling Loss

VINCENT T. DeVITA JR., M.D., AND
ELIZABETH DeVITA-RAEBURN

THE DEATH OF CANCER

Vincent T. DeVita Jr., M.D., is the Amy and Joseph Perella Professor of Medicine, Epidemiology, and Public Health at the Yale School of Medicine. He was the director of the National Cancer Institute and the National Cancer Program from 1980 to 1988. In 1988 he joined Memorial Sloan Kettering Cancer Center as the physician in chief and incumbent of the Benno Schmidt Chair of Oncology. In 1993 he became the director of the Yale Cancer Center. At the NCI, he developed a cure for Hodgkin's lymphoma with combination chemotherapy, proving that advanced cancers in adults could be cured by drugs. He shared the Lasker Award for medical research for this work in 1972. He is a former president of the American Cancer Society and a coeditor of *Cancer: Principles & Practice of Oncology*, a textbook of cancer medicine. He and his artist wife, Mary Kay, live in Branford, Connecticut.

Elizabeth DeVita-Raeburn has written on medicine, science, and psychology for many publications. She is the author of *The Empty Room: Understanding Sibling Loss*. She lives in New York City with her husband, the writer Paul Raeburn, and their two sons.

THE DEATH OF
CANCER

AFTER FIFTY YEARS ON
THE FRONT LINES OF MEDICINE,
A PIONEERING ONCOLOGIST
REVEALS WHY
THE WAR ON CANCER
IS WINNABLE—AND
HOW WE CAN GET THERE

VINCENT T. DeVITA JR., M.D.,
AND ELIZABETH DeVITA-RAEBURN

SARAH CRICHTON BOOKS

FARRAR, STRAUS AND GIROUX   NEW YORK

Sarah Crichton Books
Farrar, Straus and Giroux
18 West 18th Street, New York 10011

Copyright © 2015 by Vincent T. DeVita Jr., M.D., and Elizabeth DeVita-Raeburn
All rights reserved
Printed in the United States of America
Published in 2015 by Sarah Crichton Books / Farrar, Straus and Giroux
First paperback edition, 2016

The Library of Congress has cataloged the hardcover edition as follows:
DeVita, Vincent T., Jr., 1935–
    The death of cancer : after fifty years on the front lines of medicine, a pioneering
oncologist reveals why the war on cancer is winnable—and how we can get there /
Vincent T. DeVita, Jr., M.D., Elizabeth DeVita-Raeburn.
        pages   cm
    Includes index.
    ISBN 978-0-374-13560-7 (hardback) — ISBN 978-0-374-71417-8 (e-book)
    1. DeVita, Vincent T., Jr., 1935–   2. Cancer—History.   3. Cancer—Chemotherapy.
4. Oncologists—United States—Biography.   I. DeVita-Raeburn, Elizabeth.   II. Title.

RC275 .D48 2015
616.99'40092—dc23
[B]
                                                            2015011104

Paperback ISBN: 978-0-374-53648-0

Designed by Abby Kagan

Our books may be purchased in bulk for promotional, educational, or business use.
Please contact your local bookseller or the Macmillan Corporate and Premium Sales
Department at 1-800-221-7945, extension 5442, or by e-mail at
MacmillanSpecialMarkets@macmillan.com.

www.fsgbooks.com
www.twitter.com/fsgbooks • www.facebook.com/fsgbooks

3 5 7 9 10 8 6 4 2

The names and identifying details of some persons described in
this book have been changed.

To my daughter, Elizabeth, my son, Ted,
and their mother, Mary Kay;
my inspiration.
And to my patients everywhere.
Heroes all of them.

CONTENTS

THE DEATH OF
CANCER

INTRODUCTION

When I was a child in the 1940s, long before I had any notion of becoming an oncologist, Aunt Violet, my godmother and a frequent visitor in my household, stopped coming over. My parents ceased talking about her, too. It was as if she had disappeared. Several months into this state of affairs, my father drove me from our home in Yonkers to her apartment in New York City. He told me that she was sick and that she wanted to see me.

We went in, and I sat on the living room floor, playing with the toy car Aunt Violet had given me. The Ink Spots crooned "If I Didn't Care" from the record player. Aunt Violet was a bubbly woman, by far my favorite relative. We had a special bond. It was just like her to put on the music I loved when she knew I was coming.

I looked up when I heard the bedroom door open. The Aunt Violet I knew was vivacious, with dark brown eyes, curly brown hair, and a voluptuous figure; the woman who stood watching me was quiet, gaunt, and sad. Her skin looked yellow next to her white chenille bathrobe. I was only six, but I knew something was terribly wrong.

I knew also that I should talk to her, but I didn't know what to say. I ducked my head and began running my car around the legs of the record player, too scared and confused to look up. I was acutely aware of her standing there, silently, watching me. Finally, my father told me it was time to go home. I picked up my car, and we left. Several weeks later, my parents told me that Aunt Violet had died. She was just thirty-six.

Years later, I learned that she'd had cervical cancer. Her case had apparently been so advanced by the time she was diagnosed that there was little her doctors could do. There wasn't much that could be done for most people with cancer in those days, even if it was caught early. The main treatments were surgeries that were often disfiguring or toxic doses of radiation. Those treatments helped only the lucky few whose cancers were discovered before they had spread. There were no drugs to fight cancer then. And barely more than a third of people diagnosed with it survived.

It was such a dreadful diagnosis, in fact, that many people, including my parents, couldn't bring themselves to utter the word. If they did, it was in a whisper—"cancer"—as if there were something shameful about it. Or maybe it was superstition, the fear that merely saying the word out loud was tempting fate, like waving a red cape in front of a bull. Individuals like my aunt were the incarnation of people's worst fear: apparently healthy one minute, facing certain death the next.

Two decades after my aunt's death, as a newly minted doctor, I found my career taking an unexpected turn. A couple years after graduating from George Washington University's medical school, I walked onto the cancer wards at the National Cancer Institute (NCI), a reluctant trainee. I wanted to be a cardiologist, but Vietnam was in full swing, and doctors weren't exempt from the draft. The National Institutes of Health (NIH), which included a number of disease-specific institutes, was one of the few legal outs. It was part of the

Public Health Service, which was considered one of the uniformed services. If you served there as a clinical associate—that is, a trainee—you got credit for serving in the armed forces. I'd blown my interview for a spot as a clinical associate at the National Heart Institute. Yet I'd been offered one at the National Cancer Institute. It was a depressing assignment. But it was fighting cancer or stitching people back together on the battlefield. I chose cancer.

At the NCI, I saw a lot of people who looked just like my aunt Violet had at the end of her life. Gaunt. Sad. Yellow. In the many years since her death, neither the treatments nor the survival rate had changed much. People still whispered the word "cancer." One of my first patients told me that when he and his wife took their evening walk, their neighbors quietly slipped away, as if what he had were catching. At cocktail parties, even his friends served him his drinks in paper cups, so fearful were they that his disease, or his bad luck, was contagious and couldn't be washed off the glassware.

The study of cancer was a stagnant field, a no-man's-land populated by only a handful of doctors and researchers regarded by most of their colleagues as nuts, losers, or both. That's what I thought, too. It was what most people in the medical field believed. When I was a medical student doing my hospital training at George Washington University Hospital, there'd been just one doctor, a beak-nosed endocrinologist named Louis K. Alpert, who dared to try to do more for these patients. He was dosing them with nitrogen mustard, the first anticancer drug to be discovered, in the hope that he could kill their cancer without killing them. Nobody thought he would succeed. Most people mocked him behind his back. We called him and his medicine "Louis the Hawk and his poisons."

There were not many like him—physicians trying to extend the lives of cancer patients. More commonly, the patients were sent to nursing homes to die or told to go home and get their affairs in order. That patients might want a shot at something more was not part of most doctors' thinking. The general feeling was that efforts to cure cancer patients were bound to fail. As late as the 1960s, the respected chief of medicine at Columbia University refused to let his medical trainees make rounds on the cancer wards, lest their careers be tainted by the futility they would encounter there. This chief of medicine told the doctor in charge of this ward, the late Alfred Gellhorn, who did want to try to do more for these patients, that he was "part of the lunatic fringe."

And so it would have continued, if not for work that would soon begin at the National Cancer Institute, initiated by a handful of mavericks on the same wards where I landed as a trainee in 1963. Their research, in which I took part, led to the first use of a combination of drugs—known as combination chemotherapy—to treat and, increasingly, to cure childhood leukemia. Learning from them, I came up with a combination chemotherapy regimen for Hodgkin's disease, which cured 80 percent of people with advanced disease.

It was a first, and it did not escape the notice of a brilliant, wealthy socialite and influential health advocate, Mary Lasker, who had lost her own husband to cancer. Before long, with her unique combination of political acumen, medical savvy, and a dedicated pool of lobbyists, Mary managed to convince the president, Congress, and the nation that we were on the brink of a breakthrough and that it was time to invest large sums of money to conquer cancer.

On December 23, 1971, in front of a throng of journalists, a jubilant President Richard M. Nixon signed the National Cancer Act, which launched the war on cancer—an unprecedented federal research effort. The legislation set aside $100 million for the research, to be overseen by the director of the National Cancer Institute, who would be appointed by the president.

Today more than forty years have passed, and the country has spent more than $100 billion on the war on cancer. Where do we stand? What did we get for that huge investment? Many will tell you that we got little or nothing—that the war on cancer has been a failure, that people are still dying, and that you can't solve a problem by throwing money at it.

I say they're wrong.

I have now seen the war on cancer from every possible angle: as a researcher and clinician at the National Cancer Institute, as the longest-serving director of the National Cancer Institute, as physician in chief at Memorial Sloan Kettering Cancer Center (MSKCC), as director of Yale University's Cancer Center, as president of the American Cancer Society (ACS), and, most recently, as a patient myself. We are winning.

People still get cancer, and people still die from it. But thanks to this concentrated effort, far more people survive than was true when this war was launched. By 1990, as a result of the investments made by the National Cancer Act, the overall incidence of all kinds of cancers in the United States began to decline, as did the overall mortality rates. These figures have continued to decline every year since they peaked in 1990. By 2005, the absolute number of people in the United States who died of cancer declined even as the population was growing and aging (the risk of cancer is higher in the elderly).

Childhood leukemia is now almost completely curable. Hodgkin's disease and several types of advanced lymphomas are almost completely curable as well. Even in the case of cancers for which we don't have an outright cure, we can stop many if they're diagnosed early. We can even prolong the lives of those in whom cancers are diagnosed at advanced stages. Mortality from colon cancer dropped by 40 percent in the last two decades. Mortality from breast cancer dropped by about 25 percent. We're seeing major advances in what have long been considered difficult-to-treat tumors, such as ovarian cancer, small-cell and non-small-cell lung cancer, advanced melanoma, and prostate cancer.

The experience of having cancer is also entirely different. The brutal, disfiguring surgeries of the past have given way to less invasive operations, targeted radiation, and new drug therapies.

When I entered the field, cancer cells were essentially black boxes—mysteries. We couldn't see inside. Now, as a result of the billions invested in the war on cancer, we have a much greater understanding of why cancer happens and how it behaves, on a genetic and molecular level—an understanding that has led to a breathtaking array of new treatments, biological therapies, and chemicals targeted specifically to the patient's cancer cells. Immunotherapy, using the patient's own immune system to fight cancer, has become an established treatment. Advances occur almost weekly; medical journals are bursting with new ideas and therapies.

I believe we will see the end of cancer as a major public health issue. And we have the critical mass of knowledge to get us the rest of the way. We do face obstacles, but most of them are not scientific. Rather, they are in the form of not using what we know and the tools we already have to cure more because of a reluctance to drop outdated beliefs, bureaucratic battles among physicians and medical groups, and a Food and Drug Administration (FDA) that has not caught up with the innovations in cancer drug development.

These issues are well-known to doctors and researchers, but many are reluctant to talk about them overtly for fear that they could damage their colleagues or their chances of getting a grant or anger the powerful FDA. In fact, some of my colleagues are uneasy about my telling this story.

Not long ago, I had lunch with Jim Holland, one of the founding fathers of chemotherapy, the man who recruited the first leukemia patients to the NCI, at a little Italian restaurant down the street from Mount Sinai's Ruttenberg Treatment Center in Manhattan, where he works. Jim is now ninety, but he hasn't changed. He's still got a robust laugh and sports outrageous ties, just as he did when we were starting out.

I told him what I intended to write, expecting his usual boisterous encouragement. Instead, he got a serious look on his face. "Vince, you don't want to do that," he said. "The public doesn't need to know these stories."

I love Jim, but I disagree. I decided to write this book because I felt that the taxpayers who funded the war on cancer should know how their money was spent and that people with cancer and their families should know what is available for them—and how to make sure they get it. I want to lift the scrim that separates the public from those who study this disease and the individuals and institutions that treat it.

What you will see behind the scenes is not always flattering. The process of science is inextricable from human nature. As James Watson wisely said, in the preface to his autobiographical book about discovering the structure of DNA, *The Double Helix*, "Science seldom proceeds in the straightforward logical manner imagined by outsiders. Instead, its steps forward (and sometimes backward) are often very human events in which personalities and cultural traditions play major roles."

It's true. It will always be true. Watson's book illustrates it in the search for the structure of DNA. In this book, I show you how it unfolded within the context of the war on cancer.

Watson also wisely says that other participants in his story might tell it other ways, either because of the vagaries of memory or because they saw it differently. *The Death of Cancer* is not a comprehensive look at cancer or an encyclopedia of all the advances made to date. It is my personal take on the war on cancer. The truth in this book is my truth. Others might well tell the story differently.

My message, ultimately, is simple: Don't believe the cynics, the press, or the doubters. We are winning this war. In *The Death of Cancer*, I make the case—skeptics be damned—that we have the tools to eradicate cancer and will soon reach the day when "cancer" is no longer the scariest word in the English language. I will tell you how we can get there.

1

In the third act of *Hamlet*, as the prince contemplates his own death, he refers to the "slings and arrows of outrageous fortune." It's a lovely turn of phrase for profound bad luck—bad luck of Shakespearean proportions. The kind of bad luck that leaves the recipient blindsided by the way life has changed on a dime.

I chose part of this phrase as the title of this chapter because it struck me that cancer *is* bad luck. Simply put, it's the bad luck to possess cells that have acquired the ability to refire the dormant machinery capable of driving rapid-fire fetal growth and to have lost the ability to stop it. It is bad luck on the order of Shakespeare because, as anyone who has ever been diagnosed (or loved someone who has) knows, the impact of cancer on one's body, one's life, and one's family is nothing short of epic.

And yet this outrageous turn of fortune happens, each year, to more than a million people in the United States, more now than in the past because our population has grown and because it is older. One day you are fine. The next, there you are, with Hamlet, feeling cornered and contemplating mortality, while others go about their ordinary lives.

The writer and critic Susan Sontag, who was herself diagnosed with leukemia, once said, "Illness is the night-side of life, a more onerous citizenship. Everyone who is born holds dual citizenship, in the kingdom of the well and in the kingdom of the sick. Although we all prefer to use only the good passport, sooner or later each of us is obliged, at least for a spell, to identify ourselves as citizens of that other place."

No one embarks upon this journey willingly. It is outrageous fortune that propels us there. The story I want to tell you is about how this journey has changed—how far we have come, and how far we have to go.

The most effective way to convey this is by telling you the story of a patient. In the spring of 1996, I was standing on my back deck grilling a piece of swordfish when I heard the sliding glass door open. I looked up and saw my wife, Mary Kay, walking toward me, the phone pressed to her chest. She had a look on her face that I have come to know well over the years: someone had cancer.

Calls like this one are not uncommon. Because my career has given me a certain degree of visibility and because I have a reputation as someone who believes in giving cancer patients every possible chance, people find me.

Mary Kay mouthed the name of the person on the phone: Lee, a family friend of twenty-five years. Mary Kay and Lee's wife, Barbara, had met in an art class in Washington and had remained close friends ever since, even after we'd moved to Connecticut. Lee and I had gradually become close friends over the years. He introduced me to stamp collecting, probably the least eccentric of his avocations, and I introduced him to opera, a passion that had consumed much of my free time for years.

With pin-straight white hair that constantly fell in his face, piercing blue eyes, and round, wire-rimmed glasses, Lee looked like a middle-aged Harry Potter. He was a reflexively cheerful guy, the kind of person who refused to see the downside of anything. Share a problem with him, and he'd pace your living room, or sit, legs crossed, foot waggling, while he drummed up a solution. Lee liked solving problems, and as an economist for the World Bank he'd solved problems all over Latin America and the Middle East.

I took the phone and handed Mary Kay the spatula. "Vince," Lee said, "sorry to bother you." The call wasn't a complete surprise. Lee and I had spoken earlier in the week, after a frightening morning in which he'd seen blood in his urine. Like most people, he'd immediately feared the worst. "It's probably nothing," I'd said. "But you should see your doctor."

His doctor assured him that, at sixty, Lee was probably too young to have cancer. He told him that a host of other conditions could produce blood in the urine. And when he examined Lee, he found none of the telltale lumps on his prostate gland that might have suggested cancer. His best guess, he told Lee, was prostatitis, an infection of the prostate gland. He gave Lee a prescription for an antibiotic. And just in case, he ordered a PSA test.

PSA, or prostate-specific antigen, is made by cells in the prostate gland. Cancer cells make more of it than do healthy cells, so an unusually high level of PSA can be an early indication of cancer. But, as many people know, the PSA is an imperfect test. Because it can raise more questions than it answers and can spark unnecessary anxiety, many doctors don't use it routinely. And many men opt not to get it, including me. But given the blood in Lee's urine, his doctor thought he should check Lee's level.

Lee's phone call was to tell me that his PSA result had come back. "The doctor said it was high," he said, sounding uncharacteristically shaky. I was concerned, too. Lee's results didn't sound good. I was torn between giving him the raw truth and shielding him a bit longer. I opted for the latter. I repeated what he'd already heard from his doctor. "You'll need to have a biopsy," I said. "That's the only way to make a diagnosis. We won't know anything for sure until then."

I told him to have his doctor send me the biopsy report when it was done. I didn't tell him that I thought he had cancer. But I was pretty sure he did. It's true that an elevated PSA doesn't always mean cancer. But the higher the score, the greater the likelihood that it does. A normal PSA is under four. Over ten suggests a strong probability of cancer. Lee's was twenty-three.

Lee had the biopsy that his doctor recommended. It came back positive. The next step was to get an MRI, a medical imaging technique well suited to scanning soft tissue. It revealed enlarged lymph nodes around Lee's prostate gland—not a good sign. The lymph nodes that surround organs are a gateway for cancer cells. If you find cancer cells there, odds are the cancer has already spilled out into blood vessels; it has metastasized.

Prostate cancer can be a tricky disease to treat. Many prostate cancers grow so slowly that the men who have them will die of old age before they die of the cancer. This is one of the things that makes the PSA test so controversial. When men are routinely given a PSA test as a screening tool, these cancers can turn up. As a consequence, men who might never have been bothered by their cancers end up undergoing extensive testing and treatment for something that would never have become life threatening. One study of samples taken from the cadavers of men over age fifty who had died of other causes found that approximately 31 percent had evidence of prostate cancer.[1] Whatever killed those men had been more deadly than their prostate cancer. But if they'd been given PSA tests, they might well have been given unnecessary treatment for those slow-growing cancers.

We can't be totally complacent about the disease, however, because some prostate cancers are aggressive and quite deadly. Lee's was starting to look as if it was one of those. And there was another indication that it was a nasty tumor: the pathologist who looked at the tissue from Lee's biopsy gave it a high Gleason score. Devised by the pathologist Donald Gleason in the 1960s, this scoring system is a way to evaluate prostate cancer cells under a microscope and determine which are most aggressive. The higher the Gleason score, the worse the prognosis. A score lower than six usually means the cancer isn't too aggressive. In those cases, oncologists will often decide to withhold treatment and monitor the cancer to see whether it spreads—a practice called watchful waiting.

A Gleason score of seven to ten, on the other hand, suggests a patient will have a poor prognosis. The pathologist gave Lee's cancer a Gleason of ten, meaning the cells in his tumor appeared wild. They were large and had an unusual structure and more cytoplasm than a typical cell. More bad news. Cells with this appearance tend to behave autonomously—to have their own built-in signaling system. They are likely to grow out of control and invade other tissue. So far, all indications were that Lee's cancer was a very bad actor.

Aggressive, fast-growing cancers are difficult to track down and get rid of, but in the process of making copies of themselves, they have to disassemble their DNA for a brief time. At that moment, they are most vulnerable, and we can attack.

But we have to be smart about what we hit them with—and how aggressively. Cancer cells are cannily adaptive; they learn to outwit therapies quickly. So the first attempt to treat a cancer has the best odds of curing it, because we're hitting it with something it's never seen before. The cancer is more vulnerable and treatable than it will ever be again. This is one reason recurrences are so troubling: you're dealing with much smarter cells by then.

This was all going through my mind as Lee and I exchanged e-mails and phone calls during the week after his biopsy. Even with positive nodes and a high Gleason score, Lee had a chance—a slim one—that rested on getting that best first shot. We needed a doctor willing to try everything we had in our prostate cancer arsenal. That worried me more than Lee's soaring PSA.

When I was a young oncologist working the wards at the National Cancer Institute, we had the freedom to try anything and everything for each individual patient. We had fewer tools then, and you had to be flexible to maximize the chances for each patient. There was no prescription for how to handle a specific cancer because we were inventing it as we went along. Gradually, day by day and week by week, we figured out how to cure more people.

Over the years, we've gained more tools for treating cancer, but the old ability to be flexible and adapt has disappeared. Many doctors now rely on what are known as standards of care—treatment guidelines issued by professional organizations or government institutions. These are based on the advice of expert panels and evidence in published studies that spell out the best treatment for most patients with a particular kind of cancer. The standards of care also explain how and when the treatment should be used.

To establish these guidelines, doctors look at such things as typical responses to chemotherapy and the median survival curve—the length of time that 50 percent of patients will remain alive for a given treatment. The idea is to establish what's best for the largest number of patients. The guidelines have a big impact on care. The FDA uses them when considering drug approval, and insurance companies use them when deciding whether to reimburse patients for treatment. If a patient's treatment meets the standard of care, insurers will usually pay for it. If it deviates too far from that, insurers are likely to pronounce the treatment experimental or unproven and refuse to cover it.

Malpractice lawyers are ready to pounce on treatment that doesn't meet the standard of care, arguing that the patient they're representing didn't get the best possible treatment. As a result, doctors have strong incentives not to stray too far from the standard of care. And for many patients, this system does indeed help ensure that they will get the best treatment.

But this state of affairs also raises problems. Guidelines are backward looking. With cancer, things change too rapidly for doctors to be able to rely on yesterday's guidelines for long. These guidelines need to be updated frequently, and they rarely are, because this takes time and money. But if they're not revised to reflect advances in treatment, patients who might have been cured by newer approaches will die. Reliance on such standards inhibits doctors from trying something new.

My concern was about the standard-of-care guidelines for prostate cancer. Lee's situation wasn't well suited to the guidelines that were current in 1996. Neither surgery nor radiotherapy by itself could extend the median survival for those with prostate cancer that, in cases like Lee's, had already spread to the lymph nodes. According to the standard of care, therefore, doctors had dismissed these two forms of treatment in favor of what had worked best: administering drugs to block the naturally produced testosterone that stimulates the division of prostate cancer cells. Deprive those cells of testosterone, and you'll slow their incessant growth. For a time.

The problem was that although this approach improves median survival, it doesn't cure anyone, and everyone in the medical community knew it. All cancers are canny and adaptable. Prostate cancer cells eventually and inevitably found a way to grow, divide, and spread without the presence of testosterone. At best, this therapy, known as androgen deprivation therapy, or ADT, bought the patient a little time. As an oncologist, buying patients time is one of my primary strategies. Not so that they can get their affairs in order, or face the inevitable, but because I want to keep patients going until the next new treatment comes along so that they can take advantage of it. But Lee's cancer was so ferocious that I didn't think ADT would extend his life for more than two or three years—at best. I didn't think that was long enough to get us to the next advance. We needed more time.

I wasn't surprised when Lee called and told me that his urologist recommended that he go on ADT treatment. His urologist, I noted, hadn't told him the therapy would likely provide little benefit. That didn't surprise me either. It's not easy to deliver that kind of news, and many doctors simply don't do it. But I'm an aggressive doctor. I will do whatever it takes to cure patients and, if that isn't achievable, keep them going as long as possible. So the bigger issue, from my perspective, was whether there was something else, something better than hormone deprivation, we could try. But I couldn't make Lee's decisions for him, so I did what his urologist had not: I explained the situation and asked him what he wanted.

"Ten years," he said. I asked him what he was willing to do. "Anything," he said.

I had an idea. Clinical studies of new cancer treatments report their successes or failures in the aggregate: what percentage of patients survived for five years, say, or how many gained a few months. But a search through the details in these studies often yields clues about what might work even better for a certain minority of patients.

Not many people have the time or expertise to search for and find such clues. But I do. It's what we did in the pioneering days at the National Cancer Institute, when survival rates were low and we looked everywhere for ideas as to what to try for our patients. It's the kind of thing a determined oncologist can do on behalf of a patient now if he or she is unwilling to settle for a ho-hum standard of care.

I had heard about a prostate cancer study at the Mayo Clinic where researchers were exploring the use of radical prostatectomy—removing the prostate gland and the surrounding lymph nodes—in patients whose nodes had not yet been infiltrated by spreading cancer cells.[2] The standard operation in these cases was to remove only the prostate gland and leave these nodes, the assumption being that removing the nodes as well made the surgery more extensive without affecting the odds. There wasn't any evidence that survival could be extended by removing nodes to which cancer cells had not apparently yet spread. Why bother?

The Mayo group had discovered, however, that in about a third of cases there was undetected spread of the cancer to the lymph nodes. Nodes that appeared to be free from cancer cells were not. And the Mayo researchers were finding that removing the nodes in these patients improved survival. The researchers hadn't seen enough of an impact to justify the treatment for all people with prostate cancer and lymph node involvement. But about 15 percent of treated patients were surviving free of disease.

I found this particular number—practically a footnote in the article—to be more interesting than the researchers suggested. It was a better result than what I'd seen in most other novel therapies at that time for metastatic prostate cancer, which is what Lee had. I thought it was worth a try for him. I called the chief surgeon of the group and asked if he would see Lee. Then I asked Lee whether he was willing to make the trek to Minnesota, where he might have major surgery away from most of his family. He agreed to give it a try. Unfortunately, when doctors at the Mayo Clinic examined him, they decided that his cancer was too advanced for their study. They refused to operate.

We were down but not out. I changed course and looked for someone else who was doing this type of surgery. I found Marston Linehan, an experimental urologist who worked with my good friend Steven Rosenberg, chief of surgery at the National Cancer Institute. Linehan wasn't experimenting with lymph node surgery as treatment, but he knew how to do the surgery because of his research: He was collecting positive nodes to build a database on molecular abnormalities in prostate cancer. His goal was to see if there was a consistent mutation of a gene in prostate cancer that could be used as a target for future treatment. He was already famous for work he had done in kidney cancer identifying a driver mutation called the VHL gene.[3] This kind of work was new then, but it was the way of the future.

When I asked Linehan about Lee, he hesitated. He was deeply involved in his research, which was aimed not at helping patients like Lee now but at helping patients in the future, once he'd learned more about the spread of prostate cancer. But I can be very persuasive. I explained that Lee could provide the kind of tissue he needed. "I'm sure he'll be willing to take part in the study," I told him. "He lives right there; the NIH is in walking distance of his house."

"I'll do it if I can keep the tissue," Linehan said. That was fine by Lee. Linehan removed his lymph nodes through his abdomen, laparoscopically. Five of them were packed with cancer cells.

The next step was radiotherapy to take care of the tumor in the prostate gland itself—which had not been removed—and to destroy any cancer cells in the remaining lymph nodes that Linehan hadn't removed.

Although I'd spent a huge portion of my career at the NCI and had great allegiance to the institution, I didn't want Lee to get his radiotherapy there. Most people think cancer centers are comprehensive, one-stop-shopping cancer facilities. Whatever type of cancer you have, they can handle every aspect of it. But the truth is, they can't. Different institutions have different strengths. The NCI had once been very strong in radiotherapy, but it wasn't anymore.

I sent Lee to my friend Zvi Fuks, chairman of radiotherapy at Memorial Sloan Kettering Cancer Center in New York City. Zvi was one of the most capable, aggressive, and adventurous radiotherapists I've ever known. He was investigating some novel ways to irradiate prostate cancer. Plus, Sloan Kettering had the best equipment. I knew that because we bought it during my tenure as physician in chief there.

MSKCC also had Clifford Ling and an entire department of the finest dosimetrists in the world. These scientists figure out the precise calculations regarding the radiation dose and how to irradiate the patient without damaging organs in the vicinity of the treatment area. Good dosimetry is indispensable for safe radiotherapy. Too low a dose to the tumor will lead to relapse. Too high a dose a millimeter away from the tumor can destroy a vital organ.

Lee and his wife, Barbara, rented a furnished apartment in the Yorkville neighborhood on the Upper East Side of Manhattan for the six weeks the treatment would take. Lee walked the mile to MSKCC and back every day for his treatments, and he and Barbara walked the entire city in their spare time, exploring museums and restaurants and enjoying Broadway shows and operas.

By the time Lee had finished treatment, his PSA had become undetectable—a sign that the cancer either was gone or had been knocked off its feet. All we could do was hold our breath and wait. The plan was for Lee to have a PSA test every three months and a scan every year. If his cancer recurred, we wanted to know quickly.

The fact that he had had all three bad risk factors—a high PSA; a wild cell type, as evidenced by the Gleason score; and cancer cells in his abdominal lymph nodes—meant the cancer would probably recur.

I told him he had a high risk of recurrence, but I didn't beat him over the head with it. I wanted him to have hope, too. Even if his PSA did start to rise, I told him, we would likely have become smarter about how to handle it.

Lee briefly went back to work at the World Bank and then enjoyed an active retirement. He felt good and looked good, and his usual enthusiasm had returned.

In 2002, a little more than five years after his diagnosis, Lee's PSA spiked.

It surprised me that it had taken so long. Given the wild nature of his tumor, once it started growing unchecked, it should have developed quickly. This indicated that the tumor cells that had survived had probably remained dormant for a while, injured but not killed by radiotherapy.

Lee still felt normal, and his scans at Sloan Kettering did not reveal evidence of a tumor mass of any kind. He was classified as a "biochemical relapse"—that is, the only indication of the presence of tumor in his body was the measurement of a chemical, the PSA, in his bloodstream. The tumor he had was too small for us to measure or even see.

The standard approach to biochemical relapse in surgically treated patients was to give radiation to the tumor bed, the place from which the tumor arose, because some tumor might have been left behind. But Lee had already had all the radiotherapy he could manage. The other option was ADT, to starve the tumor of testosterone.

But it was 2002, a time when most doctors were choosing not to treat right away. They usually waited until there was evidence of visible tumor or other signs and symptoms, such as bone pain, which meant the cancer had spread to the bone. Then they would use ADT, which didn't cure anyone with advanced prostate cancer but served as a palliative to lessen symptoms when necessary. Most doctors saw hormone treatment as the slippery slope to the end.

I saw it differently. At the time, I regarded patients in biochemical relapse as the new frontier in prostate cancer treatment. It was an ideal place to test whether prostate cancer was curable by chemotherapy, because these patients, free of visible tumor, were usually in good condition and able to tolerate the treatment. What's more, their PSA level would allow us to gauge how well the patient was responding. If a treatment knocks down the PSA, it's doing something; if not, it isn't.

But at that point, we had no FDA-approved chemotherapy for patients with biochemical relapse. We didn't have a lot of studies evaluating chemotherapy after surgery in high-risk prostate cancer patients. And we had almost none using chemotherapy for patients, like Lee, with only biochemical relapse. But there were drugs around that experienced investigators felt had a significant effect on prostate cancer that could be tried. I found one lone ongoing trial in the literature for patients undergoing biochemical relapse that seemed applicable to Lee's situation. The study was looking at the use of two chemotherapy drugs, on top of ADT, for these patients.

After overcoming some hurdles, we managed to get Lee enrolled in the study. At the end of the treatment regimen, in 2003, his PSA was almost zero again, but not quite. That worried me. Back in the 1960s, when I was beginning to work on Hodgkin's disease, I learned that as long as people are responding to treatment, you must continue it until there's absolutely no sign of cancer left. Then, especially if you have no marker like the PSA to follow, you give them a couple more rounds, because even if you can't see them, cancer cells are almost surely still lurking in the system. And those cancer cells can, in short order, divide and become more cancer cells, until they've created a brand-new tumor. All patients should be treated like this; it makes no sense to stop therapy when you've got the upper hand.

But the investigators of this trial had designed the study so that each patient got a fixed number of doses—regardless of what their numbers looked like at the end of the study. To change course would require the investigator to go to the Internal Review Board (IRB) at the hospital where the study was taking place and make the case that therapy should be continued. Doctors hate going back to IRBs once a study protocol has been signed off on. It's time-consuming, it makes the doctor appear difficult to the people on the board, and IRBs, in the name of protecting the institution, the patient, and the integrity of the study, are notoriously rigid. Often too rigid.

I told Lee that he should urge his doctor to allow him to continue treatment, even though it would deviate from the guidelines of the study and even though it meant a special request to the hospital IRB. I outlined the argument for him. The doctor said no. He said he was pleased with his results and that Lee should be, too. "Maybe your body will keep responding," he told him.

I was dumbfounded. This was Lee's only chance for another long remission. Was it possible that the physician didn't realize it? Or, more likely, he figured trying to obtain a departure from the protocol would be futile. (Indeed, when I presented the case as a hypothetical to an oversight group at Yale years later, they told me that they would not have approved it.) I was angry and frustrated, but I was in a difficult spot. Lee wasn't my patient—I was acting as a consultant to a friend—and it wasn't my study. Nor was I the one who would be walking out on a limb in front of the IRB. I could use my connections and position to try to force the doctor's hand. But if I overstepped the boundaries, it could drive a wedge between Lee and his doctor, whom he admired, and compromise his medical care.

Several beseeching e-mails later, it was apparent that I was getting nowhere. I feared losing Lee for all the wrong reasons—not because there wasn't a therapy that might help, but because of bureaucracy and its attendant inertia. I thought about calling the doctor and trying a more personal approach, but given how my e-mails had been received, I thought the doctor would perceive this as stepping over the line. In the end, I didn't call. It was a mistake I would live to regret.

Lee went home, thrilled with his almost undetectable PSA. I didn't tell him how concerned I was, but I knew that he had just lost his best chance for survival. It would only be a matter of time before the cancer came back even more aggressively, and I'd be looking for the next possible treatment. And this time, his tumor would be even harder to control. Somewhere, hidden in Lee's body, I imagined prostate cancer cells having a cynical laugh. They were winning.

There was not much else I could do for him at that point but wait. I had already moved him from his urologist's hospital to three different cancer centers and had tried to come up with something else. I searched the literature again and again but found nothing. There was no other systemic therapy that had been shown to work. No amount of arm-twisting on my part would have persuaded any doctor to risk his reputation and treat Lee with anything other than ADT.

By the middle of 2004, Lee's PSA began rising again. His doctor and I agreed to get repeated PSAs, spaced out over several months, to give us an idea of how fast his tumor was growing. We wanted to know how long it would take for his PSA to double. Six months later, it was clear that his PSA was doubling every three months. His tumor was now expressing itself the way it had in the beginning. It was wild.

His doctor decided to try ADT. There was nothing else. Lee's PSA fell quite a bit, but gradually it began to climb again. At some point, most advanced prostate cancers get smart and figure out a way to grow, even with no or very little testosterone. This had now happened to Lee.

By this time, it was 2007, eleven years after Lee's diagnosis and four years since the end of the trial in which his PSA had gone almost to zero. The paper from that study now appeared in the medical literature. Forty percent of the men who had been treated until their PSA was zero had stayed free of all evidence of cancer for up to seven years, even though their testosterone levels had risen back to normal. Lee had been so close to being one of them.

But I wasn't done. In my continual scans of the medical literature, I found another possible course of treatment for Lee, an experimental vaccine and a new monoclonal antibody against a newly identified target on T cells for prostate cancer being tried at the National Cancer Institute. But within weeks, he started having side effects so severe that he couldn't continue the therapy.

Lee's doctor then moved him to a study combining two chemotherapy drugs that, since his diagnosis in 1996, had been shown to be useful in advanced prostate cancer that was no longer dependent upon testosterone. One, docetaxel, had even prolonged the lives of these patients. These drugs kept Lee's PSA in check for about a year, although it never fell below twenty.

By the end of 2008, his PSA was rising again, and there was more bad news. Lymph nodes in the back of his abdomen, the so-called retroperitoneal space, were beginning to enlarge. In addition, scans showed that he now had tumor in his bones. The disease was spreading and becoming more aggressive, and he was suffering from asthma attacks, apparently as a side effect of his treatment.

Meanwhile, I was troubled by the care Lee was getting at the NCI. Lee waited long hours to be seen and was often seen by junior doctors in training who weren't aware of his long and complicated history. He couldn't reach anyone on the phone when he had questions. I e-mailed his doctor, asking him if he would be kind enough to see Lee himself. That's when he dropped the bomb. There was nothing more they could do for Lee. Once he was off study, the doctor said, they would have to discharge him. NIH rules required them to care only for patients involved in a study.

This had always been true. When I was there, we didn't accept patients at random. We took only those we were interested in studying. But once they were our patients, they were always our patients. If they were cured, we followed them yearly. If they failed a therapy, or rather, if a therapy failed them, we followed them until their deaths. Now patients who had volunteered their bodies to be part of studies were being discharged when they were sick, sometimes near death, and facing one of the most difficult times of their lives.

"This is abandonment," I told his doctor. He said it was a rule—implemented for budgetary reasons—and that he had to follow it. To calm Lee and me down, the NCI doctors offered Lee an experimental trial of yet another new drug, one of a group known as small-molecule kinase inhibitors. Tumors need a supply of blood to grow, and this drug blocks the pathway to new blood vessel formation. This drug had never been tried in prostate cancer. It was being studied as part of a phase I study—small, preliminary tests done to determine the safety and correct doses of new drugs in humans.

But Lee developed severe diarrhea as a side effect. And the cough attributed to his asthma was getting worse. He was finally seen in the clinic, where he was told to drink a lot of fluids and come back in three weeks. This was a hell of a way to be monitoring the side effects of a new drug. After weeks of waiting for a follow-up appointment, so weak he was almost immobile, he was given bad news. They were dropping him from the study. He was very sick, and I was three hundred miles away in Connecticut.

Through a colleague, I found Dr. Manish Agrawal, a very competent oncologist practicing across the street from the NIH at Suburban Hospital. The doctor took one look at Lee and had him hospitalized. He said Lee was very dehydrated and too unstable to go home. In the hospital, Dr. Agrawal did a careful evaluation and found that what Lee's previous physician had diagnosed as asthma was in reality interstitial lung metastases, tumor cells that had grown into the interstices of the lung.

Lee's situation was now desperate. Most doctors would have been afraid to treat him with more chemotherapy, because there was no precedent for it and it might not work. And, in Lee's frail state, the chemicals might kill him. Many doctors, at this point, might have steered Lee toward hospice. He was that far gone. But Dr. Agrawal wasn't afraid to try again to buy Lee more time.

Many people will tell you that treating patients with advanced cancer is not worth it. That's baloney. When a doctor says that, what he usually means is that it would not be worth it for him. Doctors often have trouble walking in the shoes of their patients. If a patient is functional and there is a reasonable chance of a useful response, I believe that it is worth trying one or two cycles of treatment. That can take a month to a month and a half. If something good and useful is going to happen, it is usually apparent by then. If nothing happens, a doctor can call it quits. We don't lose anything by trying this. And you never know what might happen.

Dr. Agrawal wasn't sure which drug to try, but as we talked, I had another thought. Lee's cancer was behaving more like a fast-growing lymphoma than a typically slow-growing prostate tumor. Prostate cancers tend to plod along in an inexorable way, but they usually don't progress as rapidly as Lee's tumor. Lymphomas, especially the type I had worked with and cured, were fast-growing tumors. A patient could develop massive nodes in the neck in a short period of time. If we were to treat Lee's prostate cancer like a lymphoma, we would need to use a combination of drugs, and we'd have to dig deep into the arsenal. Lee had already had all the drugs that had some effect against prostate cancer. What else could we use?

I thought of the drugs known as platinum analogs, which are very useful in combating a variety of cancers. One of them, cisplatin, is part of the curative program for testicular cancer. I had helped get it approved by the FDA when I was director of the NCI's treatment division. At this point, none of the platinum analogs had been tested much in prostate cancer, but one drug company was experimenting with the first oral platinum drug, called satraplatin, in prostate cancer patients.

The drug had originally been developed by Bristol-Myers Squibb and then abandoned because the company thought it too toxic. It had been taken over by a small pharmaceutical company, and I had seen the test results. They looked interesting. But the drug wasn't available for general use; it would have to be used under an FDA escape clause known as compassionate emergency use. That meant it could be used only upon request from a physician and with agreement by the pharmaceutical company to supply it. In those circumstances, a doctor could ask the FDA to approve it for use in a single patient not involved in a study.

This was a complicated process that took up a lot of a busy doctor's time. Most doctors avoided it. The FDA didn't encourage it, either. Dr. Agrawal told me he was willing to try it. But a few days later, he called me and said he didn't think Lee would live long enough for a slow-acting oral drug to take effect. When we want fast action—which Lee needed—we usually use intravenous drugs.

We decided that because he hadn't been exposed to any of these drugs and the data with satraplatin suggested that platinum drugs might be effective, we would use one of the standard intravenous platinum drugs, carboplatin, and combine it with another one Lee already had, docetaxel, that had worked to some degree. We would have to hope that he could get some additional mileage out of the combination.

This was courageous of Dr. Agrawal. Carboplatin was not approved for the treatment of advanced prostate cancer, let alone in combination with another drug that had yet to be approved by the FDA. If Lee died from the treatment, Dr. Agrawal would likely face some difficult questions from his colleagues.

Miraculously, the combination chemotherapy worked. All evidence of Lee's lung metastases disappeared. The lymph nodes in his belly shrank and returned to normal. Dr. Agrawal sent Lee to a rehab hospital for a month to get him into shape to go home. And he planned to continue Lee's treatment.

For the first time in a long time, we had a real reason for hope. Over the course of several months, Lee's PSA, which had been hovering around two thousand, dropped below two hundred, and it stayed there. Lee got well enough to sit up by himself and then to walk around on his own. As was usual for him, he befriended the people in the rehab hospital. He got to know the orderlies who had come from countries he'd worked in when he was with the World Bank. The nurses loved his attitude and his spunkiness.

When he regained his strength, he went home—to a rented hospital bed that had been installed in his living room. He got stronger by the day. The day he got in his car, by himself, and took a ride—just to enjoy the freedom of it—he came home, glowing.

The man who had been near death was now well enough to enjoy his family. He wasn't cured, but he had time to contemplate what he knew was coming.

For the better part of a year, he felt like his old self again. He was in the eleventh year after his diagnosis. He said it was a miracle, and he rapped his knuckles on the wooden table on his deck as he spoke.

Almost a year after he had started the new treatment, I got a call. His most recent PSA showed another spike. The drug combination wasn't working as well anymore. Before long, the tumor would have outwitted it.

We would have to try something new. I began exchanging e-mails with Dr. Agrawal, trying to come up with something. I didn't know whether we had another miracle for Lee. But I thought I might find at least one new idea to try.

His doctor and I discussed a variety of options, but we both felt that we had reached the point where the side effects of cytotoxic chemotherapy agents were likely to exceed the benefits in terms of controlling the tumor. We decided it was time to stop offering him chemotherapy.

Then, in July 2008, a paper on a new drug was published in the *Journal of Clinical Oncology* (*JCO*), attracting a great deal of attention.[4] The drug was called abiraterone, and it had been used only with a handful of patients in a phase I study. But it was exciting. Abiraterone inhibited a key enzyme, CYP17, involved in the body's manufacture of testosterone. If a patient can't make testosterone, it can't drive the growth of his tumor. Because abiraterone was a drug that acted by regulating testosterone, it was particularly suited to treat prostate cancer.

All the patients in the newly published study had advanced prostate cancer resistant to available hormone-deprivation treatments. The ones who had been treated with abiraterone had gone into complete remission. All their tumors had disappeared. This would be a perfect option for Lee because the side effects were minimal. It did not damage the bone marrow. And even if it didn't work, it would not exact much of a toll on him.

I decided to call my colleagues who were working with the drug to see if they would admit Lee to their studies. But I hit a wall. Once the study in the *JCO* paper was finished, the researchers had begun a new trial examining the effects of abiraterone in patients who had less advanced cancer than the patients in the original trial. No provisions were made for providing drugs to patients with more advanced disease.

I asked people about compassionate emergency use, among them my friend and colleague Howard Scher, the foremost medical oncologist specializing in prostate cancer in the United States. Howard had seen Lee during his radiotherapy treatment at Sloan Kettering, but no one, including Howard, was able to use it off study without violating requirements established by the FDA and the company that made the drug.

Howard said he had stopped answering his phones, which were ringing incessantly. He sounded pained. I am sure it was because he had plenty of his own patients who were near death's door and who wanted another year of life. The irony here was that even though abiraterone had been found to be useful in patients with very advanced prostate cancer, none of the new studies were being done in those patients.

Much to my surprise, neither Lee nor Barbara ever mentioned the news stories about abiraterone. So I was spared the depressing task of telling them that I thought it was a good treatment option but that there was no way I could get it for him. We were at the end of the line, but not for the right reasons. It wasn't because we were out of options; it was because regulations and research protocols stood in the way.

Lee had extracted a promise from Barbara to let him die at home, and she arranged for hospice care. A hospital bed and all the necessary paraphernalia were moved into their downstairs den. The hospice nurse and Dr. Agrawal taught Barbara how to administer pain medications to keep Lee comfortable.

It was awful to watch. I kept thinking about the treatments Lee didn't get. A lot of what-ifs crossed my mind. What if I had pressed some of his doctors to continue the various treatments? Would he still be vigorous and enjoying life?

In August 2008, Lee slipped into a light coma; he lingered for two weeks. On September 11, 2008, Mary Kay came into my study with tears in her eyes. Lee's personal war against cancer had ended. He was seventy-two.

In 2010, an update on the study Lee had entered using chemotherapy for biochemical relapse was published. Of all the patients treated whose PSAs had gone to zero during the course of the prescribed rounds of treatment, 40 percent were still alive and free of disease. One or two more rounds of treatment and Lee might have been in that group.

On September 11, 2010, exactly two years after Lee's death, I got an e-mail from Howard Scher telling me that the next studies of abiraterone had been completed and that they confirmed all the early results and more. Patients on abiraterone were surviving longer, so much so that the study was stopped early. (Researchers had deemed the drug so effective that withholding it from the control subjects in the study would be unethical.) The company that made the drug announced that it was making abiraterone available to other patients who needed it, even though it was still years away from FDA approval.[5] If Lee had lasted two more years, he could have been one of them. As with the chemotherapy study he'd been on for his biochemical relapse, it was another near miss.

One of my mantras, as I've said, is that we don't necessarily have to have the magic bullet to cure a cancer. We need a treatment to keep the patient going so he can reap the benefits of the next new thing that will come along. Progress is swift. Consider Lee's case: in only two years, what was experimental therapy was on its way to becoming a new standard of care.

Lee was fortunate, because of the extraordinary efforts we made together, to have survived with an excellent quality of life with a nasty prostate tumor for more than a decade. But I can't think of him, or his case, without sadness and without berating myself for not leaning harder on his doctors.

I could have told you a story with a happy ending. I instead chose to tell you one that could have had a happy ending because it illustrates what has been, for me, a source of perennial frustration: at this date, we are not limited by the science; we are limited by our ability to make good use of the information and treatments we already have. Too often, lives are tragically ended not by cancer but by the bureaucracy that came with the nation's investment in the war on cancer, by review boards, by the FDA, and by doctors who won't stand by their patients or who are afraid to take a chance.

It is a different kind of outrageousness, one that has proved even more difficult to address than the scientific obstacles. Cancer continues to adapt and evolve to perpetuate itself. We need to adapt and evolve even faster. We have made enormous progress. We are winning. But, as Lee's story illustrates, the true story of the war on cancer is not just a war against nature but a war of us against ourselves. It has been that way from the beginning.

2

Jay Freireich answered the door clutching a pitcher of martinis in one hand and a fistful of martini glasses in the other. I didn't want a martini just then, but there was no refusing Freireich, who'd evidently already had several. He thrust two glasses at me—one for me and one for Mary Kay—overfilled them, and stomped off into the crowd, sloppily topping off glasses in his path.

It was the fall of 1963. I was twenty-eight, one of twelve newly minted doctors who'd recently arrived for a two-year stint as clinical associates at the National Cancer Institute, one of fourteen research institutes that made up the National Institutes of Health. The hub of government-funded biomedical research in the United States, the NIH was home to some of the most brilliant research scientists in the country, all of whom were engaged in puzzling out the great scientific questions of the day. The man who had just forced a couple of drinks on us was ostensibly one of them.

My path to the NCI was serendipitous. I'd gone to medical school expecting to graduate and become a black-bag-carrying doctor who made house calls in a Cadillac, like Dr. Azzari, the physician who'd taken care of my family when I was growing up. But one of my professors had asked me to be his research assistant up at the Mount Desert Island Biological Laboratory (MDIBL) in Maine for the summer.

It was there that I'd been exposed to famous researchers investigating some of the leading scientific problems of the day on marine animals, which often had anatomies that were similar to but simpler than those of humans, making them easier to study. And it was there that I'd met Dave Rall, chief of the laboratory of chemical pharmacology at the NCI. Rall was helping the NCI identify drugs that might be used against cancer. He'd been impressed enough by me that he suggested I apply to the NCI as a clinical associate when I was done with school.

It had seemed like a remote idea at the time. We'd been sitting on the front steps of one of the rustic shacks that served as labs at the MDIBL, drinking martinis made from lab alcohol out of glass beakers. But four years later, with graduation behind me and Vietnam in full swing, I remembered it. Serving as a clinical associate would count as military service.

I got in touch with Rall and applied for two spots—one at the NCI and another at the National Heart Institute. By now, I wanted to be a cardiologist. But I'd botched my interview at the heart institute. Fortunately, with Rall on my side, I got a slot at the NCI. I was lucky. There had been fifty-three slots and more than fourteen hundred applicants. I had zero interest in cancer, however. I figured it was better than getting shot at in Vietnam, but I still wasn't enthusiastic.

The party we were attending was an annual event hosted by Rall. Most of the other clinical associates worked only on the patient wards. But two of us, Bob Rubin and I, also worked in Rall's lab, trying to identify potential cancer drugs. That's why we were the only associates invited to the party. Rubin couldn't make it; he had other plans. I wished I did, too. I was nervous about making conversation with people whose names I'd come to know through their articles in prestigious medical journals. I didn't think I was up to it—especially not while holding a martini glass filled to the rim.

Mary Kay and I took a few awestruck steps inside the front door and planted ourselves just beyond the foyer, the better to survey our surroundings. Tom Frei—chief of the medicine branch, the overseer of the cancer wards, and one of my bosses—came sprinting across the living room. At a spindly six feet five inches or so, he would have been an impressive sight on his own. But he was carrying over his shoulder a woman I recognized as a lab technician. Her skirt was hitched over her head, and she was kicking her legs. Edie Rall, Dave's wife, appeared behind him, barefoot and doing a high step. She was sober enough to take in our frozen faces. "*Relax*," she called out as she danced by.

"Maybe this wasn't such a good idea," I whispered to Mary Kay.

The doorbell rang. Gordon Zubrod and his wife, Kay, came in. Zubrod was the director of the chemotherapy division at the NCI, which made him the boss of all of us. He was a stunningly conventional man. He always wore a dark suit and tie and attended church daily. I'd never seen him show emotion or raise his voice.

After the Zubrods entered the room, it suddenly grew quiet and remained that way while they mingled with the crowd. Fifteen minutes later, they pivoted on their heels, retraced their steps, and left. As soon as the door closed behind them, the noise started up again.

Across the room, I saw Freireich lumber back into view and watched as he began to lower his considerable frame onto Rall's dining room table. Freireich, my other supervisor on the wards, was also over six feet tall but stocky and barrel-chested. George Canellos, a fellow clinical associate with a knack for nicknames, had taken one look at him the day we'd arrived and, in a mock German accent, dubbed him Obersturmbannführer SS Freireich. "All he's missing are the jackboots," he'd whispered. As Freireich made contact with the table, it cracked, sending him and dozens of cocktail glasses crashing to the floor.

"Maybe we should leave," I said to Mary Kay.

Rall, Freireich, Frei, and Zubrod were now the people I worked for. They were among a handful of pioneers in a radically new approach to fighting cancer. Using drugs, or chemotherapy, to treat the disease, they were known, for lack of a better descriptor, as chemotherapists. In the larger world of physicians, and even among those who treated cancer, they were reviled.

In 1963, there were only two well-accepted ways to treat cancer: radiation and surgery. These tools were effective only against solid masses of tumor, such as carcinomas, which begin in the internal organs, and sarcomas, tumors that originate in bone, cartilage, fat, muscle, blood vessels, or other connective or supportive tissue. But they were useless in cases in which a cancer had spread and in those that affected blood cells and the immune system, such as the leukemias and the lymphomas, which are cancers of cells that normally roam throughout the body. As a result, the national five-year survival rate for all cancers combined was stuck at about 37 percent. Those who survived were the lucky minority whose cancers were diagnosed before they had spread.

Although about 90 percent of women with breast cancer presented with what appeared to be "localized disease"—that is, cancer that hadn't spread—only 40 percent were cured by surgery and radiation. The other 50 percent already had tumor cells traveling through their bloodstreams at the time of their surgery—which meant certain recurrence.

Surgeons operated on two-thirds of all new cases of lung cancer; the remaining third were deemed inoperable. Still, only 6 percent were cured with surgery. Half of all patients with pancreatic cancer were taken to surgery, but only 2 percent were cured. Most people with colorectal cancers were operated upon, but only a third, overall, were cured.

Surgeons had tried to improve the survival rate by going bigger with their operations—a tactic inspired by William Halsted, a famous surgeon and one of the founders of the Johns Hopkins School of Medicine. It was Halsted who, in 1894, developed a technique for removing breast cancers that involved cutting off the entire breast, the lymph nodes in the nearby armpit, and all the muscles covering the chest wall en bloc—that is, as a single piece.

Halsted called this procedure the radical mastectomy. He thought that cancer cells spread like soldiers marching in single file, invading whatever lay in their path beyond the tumor. The trick was to get ahead of the cancer, removing the tissue that lay in its trail. In his original paper describing the procedure, Halsted even advocated for removal of the head of the shoulder bone on the affected side en bloc—that is, as a whole—if the surgeon decided that the tumor had spread there.

Halsted's procedure lived up to its name. It was radical. It left a woman with only a thin skin graft covering the chest wall, through which her rib cage was clearly visible. Removing this much tissue also tended to cut off the drainage path for lymph channels—small, almost invisible vessels that drain excess fluid from organs, strain it through lymph nodes, and then deliver it back to the bloodstream. This blockage resulted in the additional disfigurement of a swollen arm.

Because Halsted was a surgeon of such renown, removing tumors en bloc became the standard for all cancer surgery. In fact, surgeons referred to it as "the cancer operation."

Applied to head and neck cancers by the famous head and neck surgeon Hayes Martin, it became the commando procedure, in which surgeons took the tumor, the lymph nodes, the strap muscles of the neck and the jawbone (which make it possible to speak, chew, and swallow), and even the tongue, if necessary. It was the most disfiguring operation ever invented. Patients wore special veils across their faces to hide their disfigurement.

Applied to colon and rectal cancers, it meant permanent colostomy. Applied to tumors on the extremities, such as bone cancers affecting the leg, it meant radical amputations, sometimes removing the entire femur bone from the hip on the affected side or taking off half the pelvis, too. Applied to pancreatic cancer, it became the Whipple procedure, which involved the removal of the pancreas, stomach, duodenum, spleen, and surrounding lymph glands.

Applied to cervical cancer, it became the Wertheim procedure, in which the surgeon totally excavated a woman's pelvis, resulting in not only a colostomy but also the redirection of urine flow.

In a bid to improve upon Halsted's radical mastectomy, some surgeons went a step further and created the "super-radical mastectomy," in which they opened the chest wall and took out the internal mammary lymph nodes as well.

When I was in medical school, there'd been a lot of gallows humor related to these kinds of operations. The joke was that when the surgeon wasn't sure which piece of the patient to send to the pathologist, he kept the part that blinked.

When I got to the NCI in 1963, Al Ketcham, the chief of surgery, had tacked his motto to his office wall. It read, "If you can't go wide, go deep."

The story was similar with radiation therapy. It, too, had been born in the late nineteenth century, after Marie and Pierre Curie discovered radium and Wilhelm Röntgen discovered X-rays. Soon these penetrating rays were used to diagnose fractures as the separated pieces of bone were easily visualized. At lower voltage, these rays were used to create a fluoroscope image, a kind of living X-ray in which the beam passed through the body and created an image on a fluorescent screen. Doctors could visualize organs in real time. The technique was used to detect fluid in the chest, which was common at a time when tuberculosis was rampant.

It didn't require a big intellectual leap to wonder if X-rays could have an impact on tumors if given in higher doses. It turned out that ionized elements created when X-rays hit tissue can cause damage and even cell death by breaking the DNA strands of tumor cells in two.

How well a beam penetrates depends on the energy of the beam itself, which is a function of the amount of voltage used. The original machines were kilovolt (thousand-electron-volt) machines emitting low-energy X-rays. Unfortunately, a lot of the dose never got beyond the skin. But at the high doses necessary to destroy tumors, severe skin burns occurred. The literature of the 1920s and 1930s was replete with pleas to discard radiation therapy as a cancer treatment because it was too toxic.

Radiotherapy is tricky. There is a dose of radiation that will kill every known cancer cell. But radiation beams penetrate surrounding normal tissue at the same time as they penetrate a cancer, and there is a limit to the dose of radiation normal tissue can tolerate before it, too, is destroyed. For each type of tissue, the tolerated dose is different. So for radiation therapy to be effective, the tumor in the path of a beam has to be killed at a dose that falls below what it takes to severely damage or kill the normal tissue around it.

While the strength of a radiation beam is that it can be aimed precisely, its weakness is the same as the surgeon's knife. If a few cells have escaped the edge of the scalpel, the patient will not be cured if nothing further is done. If a cancer cell is a millimeter outside the X-ray beam, it, too, will live happily ever after.

In the late 1950s, higher-energy machines, in the million-electron-volt range, called Cobalt-60 generators, were developed. These machines allowed the beam to spare the skin and do its most severe damage to the internal tumor. After this discovery, the application of radiation therapy to localized tumors really began to take off.

Cervical cancer patients could receive full doses of radiotherapy that still spared the excretory ducts of their kidneys. Breast cancer patients could receive radiation treatment postoperatively, and the thin skin grafts could be left intact.

But when, despite the improvements, radiotherapy failed to increase the cure rates, radiotherapists did the same thing surgeons did before them: they tried hitting more and more normal tissue with wider and wider beams. Or, after extensive surgery for certain cancers, such as cancer of the breast, they prescribed full doses of radiotherapy, subjecting these already mutilated patients to more toxicity without improving their odds of beating the disease.

The aggressiveness of these procedures was born of frustration. No matter how much more tissue was taken, or irradiated, it didn't affect the survival rate, which by the mid-1950s had leveled off. The problem of what to do about cells that escaped the initial tumor was a big one. *The* big one.

By the time I arrived at the NCI, it was pretty clear that cancers spread in the bloodstream and lymphatic system, not in a straight line to surrounding tissue, as Halsted had suggested. We needed another weapon, something adroit enough to navigate the body's blood vessels and lymph channels to chase down renegade cells and kill them.

What Frei, Freireich, and Rall were doing with drugs wasn't without precedent. As early as 1907, Paul Erhlich, the great German chemist, had begun to use rabbits with syphilis to test the efficacy of certain chemicals to fight infectious diseases. He thought about doing the same for cancer but was so pessimistic about the likelihood of success that he hung a sign over the door leading to the cancer lab. It read, "Give up all hope oh ye who enter." Other doctors had tried a solution of arsenic, called Fowler's solution, to treat leukemias and lymphomas, with no success.

The idea got another boost in 1943 when the U.S. Office of Scientific Research and Development decided it wanted to invest in countermeasures against the lethal gases that had been used so effectively on the World War I battlefields. It was anticipating the next world war and thought it needed better defense. Dr. Milton Winternitz, a Yale chemist who'd worked on chemical warfare during World War I, was asked to study the chemistry of phosgene and other gases and their effects.

Winternitz, in turn, asked Alfred Gilman and Louis Goodman, Yale pharmacologists, to study nitrogen mustard, a liquid derivative of phosgene gas that could be given intravenously.

Gilman and Goodman gave nitrogen mustard to rabbits and noted that the cells within the rabbits' bone marrow and lymph nodes disappeared. It occurred to them that this might be a positive when it came to certain types of cancers, such as lymphomas, which inhabit the lymph nodes. When they tried nitrogen mustard on mice in which tumors had been transplanted, the cancer went away. The idea of giving nitrogen mustard to an actual person was a tantalizing next step.

Gilman and Goodman found an ideal candidate, a man identified in the medical records by his initials, JD, a forty-six-year-old Polish immigrant who had worked in a ball bearing factory in central Connecticut. He was the patient of Gustaf Lindskog, then an assistant professor of surgery at Yale.

In August 1940, JD, feeling discomfort in the throat area, underwent a tonsillectomy. In December, he had pain under his jaw and underwent a tooth extraction in hopes of extinguishing it. But the pain didn't go away. Eventually, his doctors determined that he had lymphoma.

The doctors referred him to New Haven Hospital, now Yale–New Haven Hospital. The tumor was by now about the size of a softball. The notes in his file say that the mass was so compromising, JD could barely open his mouth.

JD underwent standard therapy for the time—sixteen doses of external beam radiotherapy. It was remarkably effective. His tumors, which included growths on his neck and clavicle area, shrank to almost nothing. A biopsy of the remaining tumor showed necrosis, a sign that the cancer cells were dying off. The doctors believed they had gotten it all.

Within eight months, however, the masses had returned. Again, JD was dosed with radiotherapy. This time, however, the tumor didn't respond. The records show that JD had lost weight and was having trouble speaking and swallowing because the tumors were obstructing his throat. The tumor had so consumed his neck and chest that he had to pivot his entire body to look to one side or the other.

The doctor's notes at this stage are grim. "The patient's outlook is utterly hopeless on the present regimen." He recommends admitting the patient to the hospital because "the end seems so near."

It was at this point that Gilman and Goodman must have had a conversation with Dr. Lindskog, because a note in the file reads that

Dr. Lindskog will investigate the possibility of treating the patient with one of "the newer chemicals, which are lymphocidal." The doctors couldn't specify the drug, nitrogen mustard—similar to mustard gas—because it was being studied in secret as part of the war effort. But that's what they were referring to.

On August 27, 1943, JD received the first of ten daily doses of "synthetic lymphocidal chemical." By day 4, he felt better, and he was sleeping and eating normally. By day 31, all of the masses were gone.

But there was a cost to the treatment. By day 16, JD's white blood cell count had plummeted. By day 25, he had required a transfusion. By day 34, the side effects were increasing. He was running a fever and had a cough, and his white count had plummeted again.

On the forty-ninth day after the therapy began, he'd developed a massive recurrence. Five days later, he received another three-day course of "lymphocidin" and experienced a short-lived response. Seventeen days later, he received a third, six-day course of lymphocidin. This time, his tumor did not respond at all.

Ninety-six days after therapy with lymphocidin had begun, JD died of sepsis—massive infection—and the constricting effects of the tumors in his neck and chest.

These doctors had learned two things—that the drug worked, and that its effectiveness was accompanied by toxicity. Nitrogen mustard did not distinguish between healthy and cancerous cells. It appeared as if the doctors had given JD more than his body could handle but not enough, or at the right intervals, to keep the cancer at bay.

This was a landmark: JD was the first person to receive chemotherapy for cancer. His doctors couldn't have imagined what they had launched. The millions of cancer patients who have since been helped or cured by chemotherapy owe a huge debt to JD—a man they've never heard of.

The possibilities raised by JD's treatment were intriguing. But word of this potentially lifesaving development didn't reach the public (or even other cancer specialists) for four years, because the research was under embargo until the war ended. The results were finally published in *The Journal of the American Medical Association* on September 24, 1946.

When the study appeared, many doctors were electrified by the obvious possibilities. If they could get to the cells that escaped tumors and treat cancerous cells loose in the system, they might be able to cure this disease. The country's most famous hematologists started to try nitrogen mustard in earnest. You could feel the palpable optimism in the early scientific publications. They thought they were on the brink of a major breakthrough.

Cornelius "Dusty" Rhoads, president of Memorial Hospital for Cancer and Allied Diseases (now Memorial Sloan Kettering Cancer Center), announced, "We are on our way to curing cancer."

Excitement, however, soon turned to gloom. In the studies spawned by the original experiments with JD, nitrogen mustard almost always worked, briefly, to produce partial responses, but the cancer always came back, and the patient always died. The disappointment took its toll. The same hematologists who'd crowed that they were on the brink of curing cancer became perpetual—and very vocal—pessimists about the use of drugs to treat the disease.

As far as most scientists and clinicians were concerned, the case on chemotherapy was closed. "Chemotherapy" and "cure" were no longer used in the same sentence. Chemotherapy was still considered for palliation, treatment that might make patients feel a little better before they died. But even in these cases, many questioned whether, given the side effects, it was worth it.

Not everyone was pessimistic. Some thought we should undertake an intensive, targeted push to screen drugs that might work against cancer, just like what had been done to combat malaria during World War II. When Allied troops in the Far East had been succumbing to that disease, the government provided the funding, and scientists had, in quick and methodical fashion, discovered new chemicals to treat malaria, such as atabrine and chloroquine, as well as new pesticides for mosquito control.

The problem was that cancer, unlike malaria, wasn't one disease.

The culprit wasn't a single pathogen. And in fact, we had no idea what caused it.

Two blue-ribbon committees—one from the NCI, the other from the American Cancer Society—had looked at the concept of a crash government program and recommended against it.[1] But the optimists prevailed—at least in Congress. In 1955, it provided $5 million and a mandate to the National Cancer Institute to set up a national screening program to identify potential new cancer drugs.[2] Kenneth Endicott, a nonpracticing M.D. who'd worked on the metabolism of folic acid, then a hot area in drug research, was appointed head of the new program.

From its inception, the cancer-drug-screening program had become a lightning rod for criticism by academics who had wanted the money earmarked for research grants instead. They also hated the idea of chemicals being selected seemingly at random to test their efficacy in fighting cancer. The program quickly became the butt of jokes.

But in truth, it was a productive program. Endicott had shrewdly entered into agreements with pharmaceutical companies that allowed them to submit chemicals whose rights they owned to be tested at the NCI. The chemicals were not identified by company or name.

For most of the previous fifty years, drug-screening research had been devoted to identifying an animal that would effectively predict which cancer drugs might prove successful in humans, but there had been no consensus on a model. To move things forward, the NCI had arbitrarily settled on one well-studied system called leukemia 1210, or L1210, that had been developed by an NCI investigator. It was a tumor that grew rapidly in mice and was thought to mimic human leukemia.

Under Endicott's arrangement, the NCI would screen the drugs provided for activity against the L1210 model at no cost to the company, and the data would be kept confidential. If a drug proved active against cancer, the company had the right of first refusal to develop it. If it did not choose to do so, the NCI could take over. By 1960, more than sixty thousand different chemicals were being screened each

year. Zubrod had recruited Frei and Freireich to the NCI and challenged them to use these drugs to cure leukemia, one of the most
formidable cancers of all.

Leukemia is a disease of the bone marrow, which is where all of
our blood cells are produced: the red cells, which carry oxygen and
prevent anemia; the white cells, which fight infections; and the platelets, small fragments of cells in the bone marrow called megakaryocytes that help blood to clot. Kids with leukemia often died of either
hemorrhage or infection because the leukemic cells would take over
the bone marrow, leaving too few healthy cells to manufacture new
blood cells. These patients required frequent blood transfusions to
keep them from becoming severely anemic.

It was devastating to watch this unfold. When I was an intern at
the University of Michigan, I was occasionally called to the bedsides
of kids with leukemia. They always looked the same, with swollen
glands surrounding their little necks and faces, and bodies puffy from
water retention because of the big doses of cortisone they were receiving. They were usually covered with bruises because they lacked
platelets, and it wasn't unusual to see them oozing blood from their
mouths, gums, and noses. The kids bled into their GI tracts, and they
often vomited blood or had bloody diarrhea. Leukemia wards were
bloody places.

Almost invariably, we interns were called upon to restart an IV
line that had quit working because an overused vein had collapsed. It
wasn't an easy job. When you tried to find one of the few functional
veins in these kids and insert the needle, the vein often oozed blood.
You couldn't see what you were doing. For the kids, that often meant
being stuck several times in a row. For the doctor, it meant causing
discomfort to an already suffering child. It was brutal all around.

One night, I was called to the room of a ten-year-old girl. Her
veins were a mess, and she was puffy, bruised, and uncomfortable,
but she was a pretty little girl with big sad brown eyes. Her IV had
stopped working, and I was asked to start another. I introduced myself,
dabbed at her arm with an alcohol swab, picked up the needle, saw her

cringe, and slipped it neatly and easily in the vein. It was pure luck. But judging by her reaction, it was the first needle in a long time that hadn't hurt. A big grin spread across her face.

"Hold on," she said as I retaped the IV to her wrist. She reached over to her bedside table, fished out a fifty-cent piece, and gave it to me. "For doing such a good job," she said. I almost cried. I looked forward to seeing her again, although I didn't know if I'd be as lucky with her veins the next time. But I never got the chance. She died a few days later. Her image is burned into my brain. I still remember her and that room crowded with her stuffed animals. This was the picture of leukemia I carried with me to the NCI.

There had been a few bright spots that were seized on by those working in the field. Two investigators—Sidney Farber, a pediatric pathologist at Harvard, and Arnold Welch, a pharmacologist at Yale— noting that the vitamin folic acid stimulated white cell growth, had an idea that antifolates—chemicals that inhibit the vitamin folic acid—might be useful. They helped develop two folic-acid-inhibiting drugs, known as antimetabolites, because they interfered with cells' normal metabolic processes.

In 1948, Farber had shown that these two drugs, aminopterin and methotrexate, could produce brief responses in childhood leukemia; the children's disease would abate or, in some cases, disappear, as would their symptoms. But the responses didn't last. All Farber's patients died, usually in weeks or months.[3]

Cortisone, a synthetic form of a hormone we all make naturally, was also developed around that time, initially for use in rheumatoid arthritis. It, too, produced brief responses. It was easier to use than the antifolates because it didn't suppress blood counts. But continuous daily use mimicked Cushing's syndrome, a disease caused by overproduction of cortisone in the adrenal glands. It caused puffy faces, more bruising, weak bones, and infections because it suppressed the immune system. Because of this, it was commonly only used in big doses in these kids at the ends of their lives.[4]

In 1951, George Hitchings, a physician turned chemist, and his technologist, Trudy Elion, developed two more related antimetabolites, 6-mercaptopurine and 6-thioguanine. These drugs, like the others, were administered one at a time and in low doses to avoid toxicity. They, too, produced only brief responses.[5]

The ultimate outcome, in all cases, was the same. The children died. Leukemia was a death sentence, a torment to the children who had it, their parents, and the doctors who had to stand by, knowing full well they were doing things that would not work, while the children slipped away.

It was in this atmosphere that Frei and Freireich announced that they planned to use chemotherapy to cure childhood leukemia, which elicited ridicule because everyone knew it was impossible. And then they'd come up with an even more radical idea than giving toxic drugs to children who were, quite literally, on their deathbeds. They decided to give the drugs in combination—two or more at a time. The medical community was scandalized. Using more than one drug at a time to treat something was, as a general rule, considered sloppy medicine. Using more than one highly toxic drug, in children, no less, and in children who were already suffering, was unfathomable.

Zubrod had enlisted a friend, Howard Skipper, to help. Skipper was a big, husky guy with a thick southern drawl and a high-pitched voice. At first, I thought he worked at the NCI, because it seemed as if he were always there. But he commuted from Alabama every week.

Skipper was a mathematical biologist at the Southern Research Institute, which was on contract to help the NCI screen chemicals for anticancer activity in the NCI's L1210 mouse leukemia model, used to test all potential cancer drugs for safety and efficacy. We couldn't take a drug, even a promising one, directly from the lab and inject it into a human. We needed to test it on an animal first and produce evidence that would justify the risk of trying the drug in humans. And it couldn't prove too toxic to the animals, either.

Leukemia could easily be induced in the mouse strain used, the

CDF1, by injecting it with L1210 leukemia cells. The mice were a good model because, in them, the course of the disease was extremely predictable. On day 1, a mouse was injected with a certain number of L1210 cells. If no treatment was given, the mouse died precisely nine days later. When the mice were treated with drugs that had an anti-cancer effect, death was postponed.

Skipper had done the experiments to determine the time it took for a leukemic cell in an L1210 mouse to double by counting the number of leukemic cells present at the time of the mouse's death. These simple tests involved sacrificing the mice, slitting them open and collecting the leukemic cells from their bellies, where the L1210 cells had been injected and grew, and counting them.

By knowing these two pieces of information—the number of leukemic cells he started with, and the number present at death in a mouse—Skipper knew how many of the leukemic cells had grown in the course of the disease from beginning to end. Then, when he gave mice that had been implanted with L1210 cells a dose of a drug, he could, by counting the number of cells present at death, figure out the exact number of cells the dose had killed. Skipper ran his experiments at the same time that Frei and Freireich were running their experiments at the NCI. He would give the proposed drugs one at a time—showing that each was effective—and then in combination, to calculate the number of leukemic cells killed by each dose of a drug singly and in combination.

From there, he'd figured out which dose and dosage schedule you needed to kill the largest number of leukemic cells without destroying the mouse's bone marrow. His work was a testing ground for what was happening on the leukemia ward. He called himself the cancer institute's mouse doctor.

What Skipper had found was this: if he used carefully designed drug combinations according to intricate schedules deduced from information he developed on the growth of L1210 cells in mice, he could cure the mice of their disease.[6]

Information bounced back and forth between Skipper and Southern

Research and the NCI as Frei and Freireich worked on their young patients and Skipper worked on his mice. And after five years of trial and error, Frei and Freireich had come up with a combination drug regimen, called VAMP, to try in children with leukemia. It was named for the four chemicals used in the combination: *V* was for vincristine, which had been isolated from a bush known as *Vinca rosea*, or the rosy periwinkle. Eli Lilly and Company had tested it for diabetes but discovered that it had anticancer properties and made it available to the NCI. *A* was for amethopterin, the chemical name of methotrexate (you need vowels to make an acronym work). *M* was for the other antimetabolite, 6-mercaptopurine. *P* represented the cortisone derivative prednisone.

I wasn't sure if these scientists were maniacs or geniuses. But most of the senior doctors at other NIH institutes had long since decided on the former. Every Wednesday, in the NCI solarium, there were grand rounds for the entire hospital, where scientists would stand at the podium and discuss their work while their peers listened and, perhaps, gave helpful feedback. Whenever Frei and Freireich were featured, it was a verbal bloodbath.

Some of the doctors in the audience would scream out interjections while Frei and Freireich talked. "This is a meat market! What a butcher shop!" I saw it happen many times. Frei and Freireich ignored them, but it was embarrassing and shocking to watch. Never had I seen doctors behave this way toward other doctors. And it made us clinical associates question what we were doing. Were we doing the right thing? Were we accessories to what other doctors were portraying as unethical behavior? How could we know? And what was our recourse?

The NIH sat on ninety-two acres of farmland dotted with trees on the outskirts of Bethesda, Maryland. With its expansive lawns and clusters of three- and four-story brick lab buildings, it looked more like a university campus than an institution. The centerpiece of it all was the clinical center, a fourteen-story redbrick building that towered over the labs.

Each floor was divided, lengthwise, down the middle by a solid wall. Labs were on one side, patient rooms on the other. A central hallway, which also housed the elevators, connected the two. The proximity of labs to patients was unusual for a hospital. But the idea behind the NIH was to bring research and patients closer together, the better to translate new ideas into innovative care as quickly as possible.

Most of the clinical associates came from the most prestigious medical schools in the country, places like Yale, Harvard, and Duke, because you generally needed the backing of a well-known professor at these places to get a slot as a clinical associate there. My medical school, George Washington University, wasn't in that league, but I'd had Rall in my corner.

Most of my peers had already been warned by their renowned mentors to steer clear of Frei and Freireich. (This was going to be an interesting feat, given that they were going to be working under their supervision.) The strong message received was that Drs. Frei and Freireich were doing something crazy, even unethical, and that young doctors could damage their careers by being too closely associated with them. They were encouraged to work elsewhere when they entered their second year and had a choice of labs in which to work. Furthermore, while Frei was thought to be merely eccentric, Freireich, in particular, was reputed to be certifiable.

It seemed, in our first meeting, that Freireich knew we had all heard about him in unflattering terms and was determined to change our minds. He talked nonstop. It was as if he were used to being interrupted and wanted to be sure to tell us everything he thought we needed to know in one sitting.

There was also an official handoff of patients by the previous year's clinical associates. Each of us was to inherit about fifty patients who would now be our responsibility. In addition to those, we would be assigned new patients as they were admitted. We would be intern, resident, fellow, and primary care doctors, all rolled into one for these people. Most of them had diseases we had hardly heard of in medical school or as interns.

During the handoff, we were pulled aside by one of the previous year's clinical associates. He wanted to pass along some information he hoped we would act on. "These guys you're going to be working for are really bad guys," he said. This associate proudly informed us that he had led a revolt of the associates against the medicine branch faculty who staffed the solid tumor service, particularly Paul Carbone, the chief doctor on the solid tumor ward, whom he described as a bungling incompetent.

Then he bragged about making rounds in a wheelchair. Within the often formal world of medicine, this was shocking. During morning rounds, the group of doctors assigned to a particular ward presented new cases and problems within those cases to the senior physician on the ward. At the NIH, clinical associates were expected to wear a clean white coat and a shirt and tie. The group would assemble and stop at the door to each room. The case was then presented by the junior doctor to the attending. Then the group marched into the room and surrounded the bed. The attending usually asked the patient a few questions and examined salient features, like lymph nodes or liver, pertinent to the case. Then the group moved on. Sitting on the bed, street clothes, no tie, a dirty coat, or wisecracking was strictly off-limits and a breach of protocol. Steve, the clinical associate who'd led the prior year's revolt and was encouraging us to do the same, had regularly appeared in street clothes, sitting in a wheelchair, which he rolled himself in from doorway to doorway, clearly making a mockery of the proceedings and daring Carbone to do something. It was the highest level of insult and one that would not have been tolerated at any of the home institutions of any of the clinical associates. But Carbone had ignored it.

One clinical associate in this earlier class was so distressed at what he saw that he refused to work on the wards at all. He'd apparently forgotten that we were part of the uniformed service, operating on a unique battlefield. Refusing to do your job on the hospital ward wasn't an option. He was reassigned to a coast guard cutter off the coast of Alaska for the remainder of his two years.

I started first on the solid tumor service, and Bob Rubin was assigned to the leukemia service. But because Rubin was trained as a neurosurgeon, he didn't feel competent caring for leukemic kids, and the senior staff agreed. That left me working on the solid tumor service and filling in whenever possible, especially on 2 East, the children's ward, which was populated with kids with leukemia.

Frei almost never came on the wards. But it soon became clear that you had to be on your toes with Freireich. I would send a patient with fever for a chest X-ray, and before I could go look at the developed film, Freireich would call me with the results. It happened all the time. Somehow, he was everywhere.

He practiced a form of take-no-prisoners medicine that often went against what we'd been taught in medical school. One of the main obstacles to treating leukemia patients with chemotherapy, for instance, was that they often succumbed to infection before we could even try to treat them with drugs. They were uniquely vulnerable to infection because cancer cells crowded out their infection-fighting white cells and lymphocytes, which control the immune system. One infection they commonly fell prey to was pseudomonas meningitis, which was quickly fatal once it set in. There was no IV antibiotic known to be able to cross the blood-brain barrier, a blockade made mostly of complex lipids that few drugs seemed able to penetrate, in order to get to the bacteria.

Freireich instructed us to get around that problem by injecting an antibiotic called polymyxin B directly into the spinal fluid intrathecally—that is, via a lumbar puncture in the lower back. This was something the label on the drug vial expressly instructed you *not* to do. The first time Freireich told me to do it, I held up the vial and showed him the label, thinking that he'd possibly missed something. "It says right on there, 'Do not use intrathecally,'" I said. Freireich glowered at me and pointed a long bony finger in my face. "Do it!" he barked. I did it, though I was terrified. But it worked every time.

When pseudomonas causes an infection in a normal patient, it creates an abscess, a pus-filled mass made up of millions of white blood cells. Leukemic patients didn't get abscesses, Freireich said, because they didn't have enough normal white cells to form one. If you saw a kid with a fever, you couldn't rule out pseudomonas aeruginosa in less than a couple of days. And once pseudomonas was in the bloodstream, it was usually fatal in leukemic kids in twenty-four to forty-eight hours. Freireich wanted us to treat it as soon as we suspected it was what we might be looking at. And, because we couldn't be sure what bacteria was responsible, he insisted we use several antibiotics at a time, to cover all possible bases.

In medical school and during our early training, we'd been taught to culture the blood for bacteria, find the exact bacterial culprit, and, only then, treat the specific cause of the infection with the right antibiotic. Treating with more than one drug, without identifying a specific cause, was not standard practice. But Freireich insisted on it. The problem, Freireich said, was that as in the case of pseudomonas aeruginosa, it took days for bacteria cultures to grow, and we didn't have the luxury of time with our leukemic patients, who had few or no white blood cells and could die within hours from an untreated infection. "We can always back away later," he said. We had to either do as Freireich said, ignoring everything we'd been taught as good medicine, or defy Freireich.

There wasn't much of a choice, really. God help you if you didn't do it within an hour of detecting a fever, because Freireich would find out. And no one wanted to be confronted by Freireich, at least not where his patients were concerned.

Once while making rounds, one of the associates, Evan Hersh, did not check a very sick leukemic patient's electrolyte and magnesium levels. It was pretty unheard of then (and even now) to measure magnesium, but Freireich had noticed magnesium abnormalities in leukemic patients on chemotherapy and was on the lookout for them, because low magnesium could lead to cardiac rhythm problems and death. Evan's patient, who was responding well to treatment, had died overnight. Freireich thought it might have been because of a low magnesium level.

He confronted Evan in the middle of the hallway opposite the nurses' station on rounds with five of us standing around. Evan tried to defend himself, saying he doubted it was the cause of the child's death. This only enraged Freireich. His face reddened; he balled his fists and brought his face an inch from Evan's and shouted, "Murderer!"

We were all shocked. Evan started to cry. It was a tense moment, but Freireich, in his own fashion, had made his point, again. You didn't give up and you never let up just because a patient had a fatal illness. We needed to give him or her every possible chance to survive. (When Freireich left for the MD Anderson Cancer Center in Houston, Texas, in 1964, Evan Hersh followed him and worked with him for twenty years. Freireich might have been outrageous, but he engendered loyalty, too.)

And then there were the platelet and white blood cell transfusions that Freireich had started trying as a means of alleviating the bleeding problems in these kids and their vulnerability to infection. Today platelet transfusions are routine for blood banks and are now a business worth more than $100 million a year in the United States. White blood cell transfusions are possible but still rarely used. But back then, nobody gave platelets and white cell transfusions because they thought it was impossible. White blood cells normally travel in the bloodstream by hugging the walls of the blood vessels. When they do that, they aren't even measurable and are called the marginating pool of WBCs. When we gave them as transfusions in an arm vein, the first organ they hit was the lungs, where they stuck to the walls and clogged the blood vessels normally used to exchange oxygen, so patients got anoxic—low on oxygen—and acutely short of breath and quite ill. In time, the cells would slip through, but the acute effect was too toxic to use regularly. No one thought they worked, anyway.

Platelet transfusions were considered an abomination. Platelets couldn't be concentrated, so you had to give them in huge amounts—about four pints. That amount in an IV bag resembled a two-foot-long sausage—a lot of liquid to filter into someone's veins. The fact that many of our patients were tiny children made it even trickier. If you gave a small volume, you gave few platelets, and they didn't work, and, worse, because platelets didn't come from donors who were an exact blood type match, they sensitized patients to the platelets, too, so in the future their immune systems would react. You had to give several million platelets per transfusion to get a measurable bump in the platelet count. In those days, that meant at least two pints.

But when you give large volumes of fluid to any patients, you can push them into heart failure because the heart can't handle pumping the increased quantity of fluid. When we were transfusing little kids who only had a couple of quarts of blood, adding a quart in a hurry would throw them into heart failure, known as pulmonary edema. The backed-up fluid behind the heart would leak into the lungs, and the kids would have trouble breathing.

Most people didn't even attempt it. But Frei and Freireich did. Freireich had worked with engineers at GE—one the parent of a patient—and developed special centrifuges that could differentially separate red and white blood cells and platelets.

So we were giving white cell and platelet transfusions successfully. But this was still verboten territory as far as our training went. Some of the clinical associates were so uncomfortable with Freireich's methods that they complained to the clinical director of the NCI, Dr. Nathaniel Berlin. Berlin was either tired of seeing these clinical associates in his office or horrified enough about the transfusions that he called Freireich into his office and told him to cut it out.

Freireich explained that while the transfusions were difficult, they had markedly reduced bleeding as a cause of death on the leukemic wards. Berlin told him to stop or he'd fire him. Freireich left his office and went right on doing the transfusions. He later told me he thought about it and decided he wouldn't want to work at a place where he couldn't save lives, so he decided to continue giving platelet transfusions. Berlin, apparently, never had the gumption to follow through on his threat.

By the time of Rall's wild party, I still didn't know what to make of what I was seeing. I admired Freireich's skills as a doctor. I even felt some kinship with him because he, too, hadn't come from an elite institution, like many of those at the NIH. I'd grown up in a middle-class family in Yonkers, New York, attended William and Mary College and a respectable medical school, although not one of the Ivies. He'd grown up in inner-city Chicago during the Depression in a tough neighborhood and in deep poverty. He'd only made it out by virtue of a kindly physics professor who'd seen some promise in him. The professor had gotten him into college, and his mother, seeing a chance for her son, had borrowed train fare he'd need to get to school and a warm coat for him, because he didn't own one. There was no doubt he was impressive, on many levels. But I still wasn't entirely comfortable with how cavalier he was about the rules of medicine.

At the party, Mary Kay and I finally retreated to a small, crowded area off the living room, hunkered down in a couple of seats in the corner, and struck up a conversation with Charlene, the lab technician who was showing me the ropes in Rall's lab. There, out of the fray, we'd found a comfortable enough place to ride out the party. I started feeling pretty good about being there.

Then two disconcerting things happened, one after another. Tom Frei strolled by the doorway, walking on his hands, his long legs in the air. (This was a parlor trick, I would discover, that he did regularly.) And Nat Berlin appeared, looking flustered. He scanned the crowd and waved me over. Wordlessly, he motioned for me to follow him to one of the bathrooms. Freireich lay in the bathtub, passed out. Berlin, a diminutive five feet six inches, needed someone my size (six feet) to help him pry Freireich out of the tub.

Together, we pulled him up, threw his arms over our shoulders, and dragged him out through the party. Berlin, mortified that a lowly clinical associate was witnessing this, kept mumbling, "We will never be able to make rounds with the clinical associates again."

Out front, Freireich's wife, Deanie, sat behind the wheel of their car. We tossed Freireich in the backseat and slammed the door. Deanie gunned the engine and took off.

The next morning, Sunday, as I stepped onto the wards at 7:00, still bleary-eyed from the night before, I caught sight of a huge white-coated figure stalking down the hallway in front of me. Freireich was already making rounds.

And so it went, day in and day out. We were there at 7:00 to draw blood from our patients and take the samples to the lab. All of our patients were on complex and intensive chemotherapy, which meant that their blood counts would be low. We needed to know how low, early, so we could arrange for transfusions if necessary. Once the labs were done, we made rounds on our patients, checking each one for signs of infection or bleeding.

We had to follow what was going on in the bloodstream and the bone marrow on a regular basis. Normal bone marrow, the factory for all the blood cells, is easy to recognize. You see large bubbles of fat, with the cells that give rise to blood cells scattered among them—big megakaryocytes, which are ten to fifty times larger than the average red blood cell and have such a large nucleus that they look like goose-berries, and smaller precursor, or blast, cells that give rise to the white cell and red cell lines.

In leukemia, the marrow is replaced by a monotonous sheet of leukemic cells that all look the same. Seeing what was in the bone marrow—whether healthy cells were regenerating and how many of them there were—would let us know if the leukemic cells were going away and being replaced by normal cells.

Every day, I had the unpleasant task of doing bone marrow aspirations. You stuck a good-sized needle into the back of a pelvic bone and retrieved a marrow sample. No matter how much local anesthesia you used, it hurt the moment you sucked up the marrow into a syringe. The pain came from the marrow itself, which couldn't be anesthetized, as the suction pulled apart the marrow structure. The kids hated it. So did I.

At the end of each day, I would take the bone marrow slides to the pathology lab to be read by George Brecher, an internationally known hematopathologist. He was among those who despised Frei and

Freireich. Brecher would take my slides, slip them under the microscope, and, with one eye on the slide, begin ranting about the crazy people I worked with as I stood silently by, waiting.

Working on the children's cancer ward was trying. No amount of medical school training or internship experience could have prepared us for it.

The children's ward was on 2 East. It was government issue, like the rest of the hospital—a blend of light-green walls and dark-green tiles. But here, the walls had been papered with kids' drawings, and there were toys scattered around the floors of the rooms. They were lovely kids, and it was hard to resist stopping in the midst of what you were doing to play for a few minutes.

Sometimes I'd be down on the second floor, goofing around with a kid in the hall, and we'd hear a respirator stop somewhere on the ward. Some people wouldn't have even noticed the sound. But I knew what it meant, and so did these young patients. As often as not, the child would look up at you, knowingly, for an instant, then look down, and resume playing. It was unnerving and sad.

There were cases, images, that became indelibly burned into my brain. A beautiful five-year-old girl whose father bolted when she was diagnosed. Her mother refused to leave after visiting hours and slept on a couch in the solarium. The nurses called me and told me to get her out, but I let her stay.

A boy whose parents couldn't leave their jobs in West Virginia and whose grandfather, who always wore a big, floppy cowboy hat, came to stay by his side. Soon after the boy died, I saw the old man in the solarium, head bent, his hat resting against a pillar.

But amid all the sadness, I saw some kids, maybe one out of four, whose disease would go into remission. They didn't die; instead, they were able to go home.

When I arrived, one of my assigned patients, a young teenage girl, was on a respirator, unable to move or even breathe on her own. She'd been given what we would now consider a huge overdose of vincristine as part of the VAMP regimen. As was the case with JD in the first chemotherapy with nitrogen mustard, no one quite knew how to use vincristine yet. Its main side effect was nerve damage, and it could cause leg muscle paralysis and foot drop. This girl had been given such a big dose that the nerves to her respiratory muscles had also been paralyzed. Freireich had her put on a respirator. Along with the other clinical associates, and even the nurses, I was shocked that she was being kept alive.

Every day, I had to tend to her fluid balance and respiratory care. Critically ill people's fluid intake and body salts like sodium and potassium often get out of balance. If left untended, they can die because of it. Then she developed pneumonia, which, given her other problems, might have led even some intrepid doctors to let her go. But Freireich insisted I treat her with antibiotics. She pulled through but was still paralyzed.

We all thought she was the living dead. It was the talk of the coffee room for weeks—the girl with leukemia who had essentially been killed by an overdose but was still alive. Barely. We wondered if Freireich was just covering his ass, keeping her breathing on the respirator. But he hovered over her and us, making sure no one involved in her care let her go.

One day, her vital signs started looking better. Soon after, she wiggled her toes. Finally, she took a breath on her own. Over the next couple of weeks, she recovered and left the hospital in a complete remission from her leukemia.

The nurses had a party celebrating her discharge. All of the clinical associates attended, and so, of course, did Freireich. He didn't say a word. But the look on his face was angelic.

I was moved by this girl's recovery, but shaken. Virtually everyone else in the hospital thought that giving up on patients like her was the humane thing to do. Had it been up to me, I would have pulled the plug on her long before. We learned from her that even very severe vincristine nerve damage is reversible. And I learned a profound lesson from Freireich: never to give up on anyone.

Every day, I was still making forays to Brecher's lab with bone marrow samples from the kids we were treating with VAMP. The results indicated that the leukemic cells were disappearing and that, even while the chemo was still in these kids' bloodstream, the bone marrow was filling up with young white cells and megakaryocytes. More kids were going home.

I had to admit that Frei and Freireich were onto something. I realized that I was no longer on the fence, that you could not ride fences, in fact, if you were going to be a real doctor to your patients. To dedicate yourself to helping people survive, especially to survive this disease, you had to be an eternal optimist and very aggressive, like Freireich. You couldn't worry about what the truth was supposed to be or what you'd been told it was. You had to go with what you witnessed yourself.

Who was George Brecher to call the leukemia service a butcher shop even while, quite literally, seeing the evidence of recovery magnified before his eyes? Or Nat Berlin, who never stepped onto the wards, to prohibit platelet transfusions, when they were working? Why make fun of Jay Freireich, one of the most dedicated physicians I had ever encountered? Or Frei, who, in addition to having great vision, had the wherewithal to know how to protect the likes of Freireich from the establishment? Why should I doubt them?

Frei and especially Freireich had made me a believer. At some indefinable point in those first few months, between the bacchanalia of Rall's party and a rant from Brecher, I'd crossed a line. To hell with black bags and cardiology, I thought. I'm going to be a chemotherapist.

3

MOMP

In hospitals across the country, most children with leukemia were getting one drug at a time for as long as they could tolerate it, getting no platelets, and dying a gory death. There was no experimentation. Even the most vocal advocate for childhood leukemia treatment and research, Sidney Farber—the Harvard pathologist famous for developing methotrexate, one of the most successful chemotherapy drugs ever discovered and one of the drugs in Frei and Freireich's VAMP protocol—was dead set against combination chemotherapy.

Farber was the only real voice in favor of cancer research and care in the Harvard academic environment. He also testified frequently before Congress about the need for more research on cancer and had helped to raise millions of dollars for that cause. But like all doctors, he had been schooled to believe that combining antibiotics, or any other drugs, was sloppy medicine. He felt he was being a meticulous investigator by doing things one at a time. Because he was so prominent, and Harvard was so influential, this had set the tone for all other institutions.

Meanwhile, led by Frei and Freireich, the leukemia group at the NCI, both egged on and protected by Zubrod, ignored all that. The group working on childhood leukemia had their own meetings on Friday afternoons. Here the clinicians, biostatisticians, pharmacologists, and anyone who had anything to do with the drug protocols gathered in a conference room to troubleshoot VAMP and the other new regimes under consideration. VAMP had just been started the previous winter, and only a handful of patients had gone on the protocol.[1]

The room measured about twenty by twenty, and each wall was covered with a blackboard, rendering the space frontless and backless. It had been built by Lou Carrese, the NCI's planning officer, for devising the NCI's linear array and decision network, the systems used to evaluate potential anticancer drugs in its screening program. The linear array was a visual display of all the hurdles drugs had to overcome before they could move on. When Lou had the chalk, he'd diagram the process, and it would take him completely around the room. This was how we reduced the vast number of drugs screened each year to a few hundred that seemed to warrant more study.

In a typical meeting, people were crammed in the room, initially facing the wall opposite the door, and then everyone shifted position as we moved on to the next blackboard. Someone would present new data about something we were working on, and then people weighed in with their ideas. Chalk dust hung in the air, as did a fair amount of cigarette smoke, this being the era before anyone realized what smoking could do to you.

It was like central command or a war room. Discussion was intense, heated, and loud. It wasn't uncommon for someone to run to the board, grab the chalk from whoever was in the midst of using it, and add his ideas to the mix. Cacophony reigned.

When I got there, VAMP was the main subject of discussion. How could we make it work better? When changes were agreed upon, they were put into practice the next day. Some aspect of VAMP—dosage or the interval of treatment, say—changed from week to week, all in an attempt to make it more effective. When the changes appeared to work well enough to improve response, the approach took on a new name. VAMP eventually became POMP (same drugs, different initials, different doses and schedules). Then it changed to BIKE, this time named for some novel changes in the schedules of drug cycles used (hence BIKE, for cycling) based on some experiments done on mice.

Clinical associates weren't really invited to these meetings but could come if they liked. I used to bring two of my closest friends among the associates, Jack Moxley and George Canellos, just to gawk. Moxley was outgoing and ambitious. Canellos was an American but was such an Anglophile that he spoke with what almost seemed to be an English accent. And he had a wicked wit. They both loved it. We clustered together in a corner, shifting slightly as the group turned to the next blackboard so as to stay in the back, while Canellos sotto voce heckled Freireich and Paul Carbone, Freireich's counterpart on the solid tumor ward. "How would you know?" he would mutter through clenched teeth. "These guys are certifiable." "In your dreams." Moxley pitched in here and there, too. Their comments were audible enough but ignored. Canellos, with his penchant for nicknames, labeled the meeting "the Society of Jabbering Idiots."

At first, I was more attuned to the odd behavior of my superiors than to what they were saying. But gradually, as I found myself being won over by Freireich and what was occurring on the leukemia ward, I increasingly paid attention. Week by week, the main players in the room were adjusting their thinking and their protocols, depending on the most recent data. It was exhilarating to be around people who were optimistic enough to talk about possible cures and doing something to discover them. I had never heard cancer discussed this way.

One of the people who intrigued me most at these meetings was Howard Skipper. He held the chalk in one hand and an ever-present cigarette in the other. Skipper was responsible for at least half the smoke in the room.

It was the fall of 1963, and I was still working on 2 East, the leukemia ward, and 12 West, the solid tumor ward. And while I was generally doing the same thing on both—treating cancer with drugs—the difference between what was happening on these wards was striking. On 12 West, there was no sense of mission, unlike what you felt on the leukemia ward. On 2 East, patients were surviving. On 12 West, no one was.

The patients on 12 West tended to be older. And they had a variety of cancers—melanoma, the most deadly form of skin cancer, brain cancer, and chronic myeloid leukemia, an adult leukemia that started out chronic but, within four years, turned acute and was always fatal. We also had a smattering of patients with cancer of the breast, colon, and pancreas, as well as some with lymphomas and Hodgkin's disease, another form of lymphoma. These lymphoma patients were often uncomfortably close in age to the clinical associates.

They all had very advanced disease, and all the existing treatments had failed. Patients were there because word about the drug testing we were doing was getting out. There were some doctors who, pressed by desperate patients for something, anything, to try, were only too glad to refer them to us. There were also doctors who only referred patients to us when they had run out of insurance benefits. We were the end of the line.

Most of the studies we were doing were phase I trials, which were meant to assess what dose of a drug patients could tolerate within the bounds of acceptable toxicity—that is, how much we could give someone without killing him. It was called finding the maximum tolerated dose, or MTD. Once we knew the MTD for a new drug, we could move on to phase II, in which we treated specific cancers with what we thought were the optimal doses and schedules, to see if the drugs actually worked to treat the disease.

Usually, they didn't. Only one in fifty thousand drugs screened for anticancer activity made it to phase I testing in the first place. Only about one in five thousand of those was both effective and tolerable enough to make it through phase I to phase II. Of those, only about one in fifty went on to be of some use. Most of the time, you didn't see any useful effects in phase I, just side effects.

The response rate in phase II studies was better but still very low. The drugs were not used in combination, as they were on the leukemia ward, but one at a time. The patients were generally hopeful, unlike the clinical associates who worked on the ward.

It was dull and dreary work for those assigned to 12 West. Getting clinical associates to give chemotherapy was hard. Giving toxic drugs without expectation of anything good happening—to people who were desperate and who would shortly die—was depressing. What was needed was a leader who could convey a sense of mission.

Paul Carbone, who oversaw the running of 12 West, was a nice guy, but he wasn't the right person for the job. He was heavyset, just under six feet tall, with jet-black hair, swarthy skin, and horn-rimmed glasses. He walked with a slight shuffle and looked off to the side when he spoke to you. He tended to talk in incomplete sentences, which gave the impression that he was shifty and lacked confidence. While he knew cancer and was a competent doctor, he was unskilled at the day-to-day challenges that the clinical associates encountered on the wards, like maintaining electrolyte balance and coping with cardiac problems. It frustrated the clinical associates, and he had a hard time motivating them to perform. Because of this, it was Carbone, not the more radical Freireich, who tended to get the most blowback from the associates. Zubrod was the big boss, and Frei was below him. Carbone reported to Frei. When Frei would send instructions to us through Carbone, Moxley and Canellos called him a "messenger boy" to his face. Speaking to a senior physician that way, in any other place, was unheard of.

When I wasn't on the wards, I was in one of the pharmacology labs, tucked away on the research side of 6 North, where the acrid smell of animals—mice, dogs, guinea pigs, and monkeys—filled your nostrils and made your eyes water. Rall had assigned me to Vince Oliverio's lab. At about 160 square feet, the size of a small living room, it was a tight fit for three people. The middle of the room was entirely consumed by a marble-topped lab bench with metal sinks embedded in it and a central rack for beakers, flasks, and pipettes. Side benches for sinks and more equipment lined the wall. There were small desks on the back wall for Vince and Charlene, his lab technician, and a cubbyhole for me in one of the side benches. I could sit on a stool at the lab bench and swivel around and enter data in the lab books on my desk.

When I'd first arrived, I'd been intent on keeping a safe distance from chemotherapy. I'd asked Rall if I could work on the pharmacology of the heart drug digitalis rather than on cancer drugs. He was amused. "Sure," he said. Rall already knew what I had yet to learn—that the pharmacology of cancer drugs was far more interesting.

The cancer drug program had cast its net a lot wider since nitrogen mustard was discovered, and it was churning out a variety of synthetic chemicals for human testing, including a class of drugs known as nitrosoureas. We also had a separate branch designed to search for anticancer activity in natural products. The scientists collected plants and undersea animals for this purpose, even going so far as to isolate bacteria from the grave sites of people who had died of cancer to see if they produced more effective antitumor antibiotics. Among the potential success stories to come from the natural products branch so far were vincristine and vinblastine, already in use on the leukemia wards, and the antimetabolite arabinosyl cytosine, which came from the sea sponge *Cryptotethya crypta*, found in the Caribbean.

Once I'd given up on digitalis, Rall asked me to work on BCNU—1,3-bis(2-chloroethyl)-1-nitrosourea—which had been designed by chemists in the drug development program at the Southern Research Institute. They'd rigged it to be soluble in fats, or lipids. The hope was that when you gave it intravenously, it would cross the blood-brain barrier and get to tumors in the brain.

It had been assigned to another clinical associate first, but he hadn't gotten very far with it. BCNU was combustible. Standard procedure for potentially flammable chemicals was, obviously, to treat them damn carefully. For some reason, the other associate hadn't been particularly concerned about this. He'd taken to storing a supply of it in the trunk of his car. One day, a bottle had exploded. That was the end of BCNU for him.

"Maybe Rall is trying to kill you," Canellos said, when I told him about my new assignment. I took no chances. I mixed the drug, at arm's length, under an exhaust hood where we handled the most noxious chemicals. If the image of my colleague's blown-out trunk wasn't enough to remind me to be careful, I had only to look at the corner of the exhaust hood, where Oliverio had clamped a long, thin, upsidedown canister to a ring stand. The container had held phosgene, from which nitrogen mustard had been derived. Oliverio had put it there as a reminder of where anticancer drugs had come from.

One day, despite my precautions, I managed to spill a few drops of BCNU on my hand. The skin on which it had splattered immediately tanned. My fellow associate Phil Frost and I watched the spots closely. Me, because I was feeling slightly panicky about the drug's potential toxic side effects; Frost, because he wanted to be a dermatologist. He sniffed the potential for a self-tanner. (In the end, he decided the risks outweighed the benefit.)[2]

One of the tasks, when evaluating a new drug, was to see how it was metabolized by the body. We needed to know how much was absorbed, where and how it was excreted, and, ideally, how it worked. That meant you had to collect not only blood samples but everything someone excreted.

We had some BCNU that had been tagged with a piece of a molecule containing carbon 14, a radioactive material. After we gave it to patients, we could track its movement in their bodies. This meant that blood, urine, spinal fluid, and fecal specimens had to be collected from all the patients who received it. This job fell to me.

Collecting blood and spinal fluid was a matter of needles and vials. Urine specimens were easy enough to obtain. But fecal samples were another matter. We had to have the NIH metal shop build a special toilet seat with a detachable paint can positioned underneath. Once a day, I made "can rounds" on the ward, detaching them from the toilet seats and carting them back to the lab for analysis.

It was not the most pleasant job. Especially because, when I went to make collections, Canellos and Moxley deliberately loitered in the hallway, cracking jokes as I walked in and out of patient rooms, looking like a milkmaid with a can of feces in each hand. "Oh, look," Canellos would chortle. "Vince is out collecting his honey buckets!"

My head was full of ideas. On the leukemia ward, I continued to witness miracles. Thanks to VAMP, antibiotics, and platelet transfusions, kids who would have been dead anywhere else were getting better and leaving the hospital. And one Friday, at a meeting of the Society of Jabbering Idiots, Skipper mentioned something that got my attention. Cancer drugs, he said, killed a constant fraction of cells per dose, not a fixed number. If a drug killed a fixed number, life would be easier: you could find a dose that killed all the cancer cells. It did no good to kill *almost* all the cancer cells in an animal or, he surmised, in a human. "If you kill ninety-nine percent of a billion cells," he said, "you still have a million cells left." That was more than enough to rebound and kill someone.

To exact a cure, he said, you needed to kill every cancer cell. Then he talked about something he called "the inverse rule," which turned out to be shorthand for "the invariably inverse relationship between cell number and curability by chemotherapy." The more cancer cells you had at the start of treatment, the less the likelihood of curing the disease with drugs. Listening to Skipper's comments on the inverse rule, I realized there was another way of phrasing it. The fewer the cancer cells, the easier it was to treat with chemotherapy. And that's when it clicked: Hodgkin's disease. One thing I knew was that if you looked under the microscope at the lymph nodes taken from Hodgkin's patients, the malignant cells were surrounded by infection-fighting white blood cells, lymphocytes, and other cells associated with inflammation. The cancer cells were actually in the minority. This meant that unlike other malignancies, a swollen gland in a Hodgkin's patient was mostly due to the collection of normal inflammatory cells that had congregated there.

It occurred to me that even when a patient had advanced disease, the actual number of cancer cells was probably relatively small. If what Skipper said was true—and I had no reason to doubt him—Hodgkin's disease might be a ripe candidate for chemotherapy.

All second-year clinical associates had to come up with a project. I already had plenty of projects because Dave Rall's clinical associates worked in the lab for three months in their first year, but Moxley and Canellos were looking for things to do. After watching the grim state of affairs on the solid tumor wards, I knew that I wanted to apply combination chemotherapy to solid tumors. But I needed to pick a cancer to focus on. Skipper's comment had immediately turned me toward Hodgkin's. I mentioned it to Jack Moxley, and he was interested, too. It turned out that prior to coming to the NCI, we both had been deeply affected by Hodgkin's disease patients.

The disease was first described in 1832 by Thomas Hodgkin at Guy's Hospital, London.[3] He saw six patients with an unusual distribution of swollen lymph glands in their necks and enlarged spleens. It was at a time when lots of things caused swollen glands, but Hodgkin was sure that he was seeing something new. He wrote a paper about his observations, preserved tissues from the patients, and went on to other things.

Until the turn of the twentieth century, the assumption was that Hodgkin's was a form of tuberculosis. It wasn't an unreasonable assumption. One subtle aspect of Hodgkin's is that even patients with early-stage disease are susceptible to infections, particularly tuberculosis and fungal infections. Ergo many patients with Hodgkin's also had tuberculosis, which was nearly epidemic in the early nineteenth century. One well-known pathology textbook dating to 1919 said, "Tuberculosis follows Hodgkin's disease like a shadow."

It wasn't until 1902 that Drs. Dorothy Reed and Carl Sternberg at Johns Hopkins University, aided by microscopes, were able to look at cells that came from the lymph nodes of people with Hodgkin's. Most cells, even cancer cells, have just one nucleus. Reed and Sternberg saw something unusual—a cell with two, looking back at them like the eyes of an owl.[4]

It was Reed and Sternberg who reclassified Hodgkin's as cancer. The owlish-looking cell came to be known as the Reed-Sternberg cell. (In medicine, first spotters get naming rights. The disease was named after Hodgkin, but Reed and Sternberg had been the first to spot the cell.) Not all malignant cells in Hodgkin's look like Reed-Sternberg cells. But in order for a lymphoma to be classified as Hodgkin's, they have to be there.

Hodgkin's starts out as a solid tumor in the lymph nodes in the neck or chest and spreads to the lymph node chain next to it, and the one next to that one, and so on—in much the way Halsted had once thought all cancers spread—until all the lymph nodes in the body are involved, including the spleen, which is really just a very big lymph node. As the disease advances, the malignant cells invade the bloodstream and settle in all of the major organ systems. Eventually, all the masses are made up of Reed-Sternberg cells or their relatives.

The disease wasn't a good candidate for surgery. But you could treat it with radiation, at least in the early stages, because the way it spread was so predictable. Henry Kaplan, one of the great radiotherapists in the field, liked to say that if you wanted to learn how to treat Hodgkin's disease, you had to learn to think like a Reed-Sternberg cell. After radiotherapy, patients were usually treated with daily doses of either chlorambucil or cyclophosphamide, oral versions of nitrogen mustard. The drugs helped briefly, but they weren't enough. Eventually, the bone marrow of these patients petered out, and the tumor advanced enough to kill them. Even with the predictable spread of the disease and a couple of drugs to throw at it, Hodgkin's was generally considered incurable.

Just as I'd arrived at the NCI, a paper had come out in the *British Journal of Cancer* titled "The Cure of Hodgkin's Disease" that had caused a small commotion in the field, largely because of the hubris of its authors in using the word "cure."[5] Dr. Eric Easson and Marion

Russell, a statistician, both from Christie Hospital and Holt Radium Institute in Manchester, England, said they'd deliberately chosen the dramatic title because they thought there was too much pessimism surrounding the disease.

In the paper, they said that if patients presented with very early disease and were treated with radiotherapy not only to the lymph nodes visibly involved but also to apparently uninvolved nodes close by, about a third could live a normal life span. Vera Peters, a Canadian radiotherapist, had pioneered the technique. Easson and Russell were among the first radiotherapists to use it, and it seemed to work. The problem was, not many people were diagnosed early. In the beginning stages of the disease, patients weren't very symptomatic, or not in a way they'd attribute to cancer. They might have a swollen lymph node or a cough. They might have cyclical fevers, known as Pel-Ebstein fever, or be more susceptible to infections. But these symptoms were either vague and easy to ignore or they were attributed to something else. As the disease became more advanced, the symptoms might become more pronounced and alarming. Then the patients would be examined by their doctors—at which point Hodgkin's was discovered. Even if Easson and Russell were correct, only about 10 percent of all cases were curable by radiotherapy. They were talking about 30 percent of that 10 percent.

We needed something more for people with advanced disease. Given Skipper's inverse rule, I reasoned, that might mean we had a shot at curing Hodgkin's, even advanced Hodgkin's, with combination chemotherapy. It was worth a try. The same old treatment wasn't getting us anywhere.

I knew this all too well. Robert Morse, the Hodgkin's patient who'd made an impression on me, was still alive, but he was running out of options.

I'd first met Morse while I was training at Washington's DC General Hospital. He'd already been diagnosed and treated with radiotherapy. One weekend, his roommates had noticed that he seemed out of it and was running a fever. They'd called an ambulance, which had brought him to DC General. It turned out he had pneumococcal meningitis. It was an unusual diagnosis in a young person, but not for someone with Hodgkin's. Fortunately, the attending physician was Monroe Romansky, an infectious disease expert and the guy who had first used long-acting penicillin. Because of Romansky, we did all the right things—took a spinal tap and blood cultures to identify the infection and administered the long-acting penicillin. The mortality rate for pneumococcal meningitis was very high, but we saved Morse.

From then on, Morse was my patient. When he recovered enough to talk, we realized we had things in common. He was my age, and he was also a doctor in training, though he wanted to be a psychiatrist. When I'd gone to the NCI, he'd followed me there. He'd already had radiation. So we'd treated him with one drug and then another. It had set the disease back a bit but not gotten rid of it. He knew he was going to die.

Morse was tall and slender with short, sandy-colored hair, gray eyes, and a serious look. Every week he came to see me at the NCI, always clad in a sport coat and a tie. And every week, I'd give him either chlorambucil or cyclophosphamide. Sometimes I adjusted the dose. None of this took more than a few minutes. But he always quizzed me. He wanted to know why I was giving him a drug, the details about how it worked, and the side effects.

But mostly, during his appointments, he wanted to talk about what it was like to die as a young man. I was uncomfortable at first. Medical school doesn't prepare you to speak with patients about their impending deaths. And even though I was now compelled to deal with death quite a lot, I hadn't gotten past my discomfort. But Morse told me he needed to talk, that it helped him deal with it. Mostly, I listened. Sometimes he pressed me for answers I didn't want to give. "How do patients with Hodgkin's die? What's it like? Is it painful?" I tried to avoid answering, but he pushed for details. He wanted to know.

Robert's youth wasn't unusual. The average age for diagnosis with Hodgkin's is thirty-two. I was twenty-eight, and so were most of the other clinical associates who'd gone to medical school right after college. You couldn't see a patient with Hodgkin's without being uncomfortably reminded that these things can, and do, happen to people just like you.

To try combination chemotherapy on patients with Hodgkin's, Moxley and I needed to develop a regimen and get Frei's approval. Overall, I felt pretty good about how I was doing at the NCI. In fact, my gritty training at DC General had actually given me a bit of an advantage. While my peers who'd attended elite programs had been exposed to famous professors who told them about various situations and diseases, they'd received little or no hands-on training. At DC General, while you didn't have the elite professors, you were pretty much always overwhelmed with very sick patients. You had to learn to handle acute problems on your own, like reading EKGs and managing electrolyte balances, because there often wasn't time to call in someone else, and sometimes there was no one else to call. As a result, I could handle procedures and situations that none of the other associates could. At the NCI, I walked around with a special three-headed stethoscope that was good for diagnosing heart murmurs, and I was the go-to guy when murmurs were suspected.

Even so, I wasn't entirely sure of myself yet and was glad that Moxley and I were on the same page with regard to Hodgkin's and combination chemotherapy. It was too far out on a limb to go on your own. And if I was going to dangle out there, Moxley was a good guy to have along. He was a good-looking, take-charge, well-spoken kind of guy with a quick, melodious laugh. And he knew exactly what he wanted to do professionally. When I first met him, the day we'd all arrived for training, we shook hands and asked each other the usual questions, including "What are you going to do after this?" Moxley's response was "I want to be a dean."

I was taken aback. Becoming dean of a medical school was something you did at the end of your career, after you were done with practicing medicine or had an academic career and you'd exhausted all the other job opportunities. No one started out wanting to be a dean.* The clarity of his vision was striking, given that I had arrived at the NCI not so much to further my career as to avoid Vietnam. It was not much of a plan.

But we'd quickly become close friends. In the first few months at the NCI, when I was still thinking about becoming a cardiologist, I'd discovered that the Georgetown School of Medicine, ten miles down Wisconsin Avenue from the NIH, had an excellent cardiologist, W. Proctor Harvey, who hosted an unusually good Thursday evening conference. It was held in Georgetown University Hospital's auditorium, which had audio equipment capable of playing heart sounds and murmurs. Harvey was the guy who had designed the three-headed stethoscope I wore around my neck at the NCI. I loved his lectures, and I'd cajoled Moxley into going with me every week. Afterward, we'd go have a few beers at the Lehi Grill, a dark, friendly little restaurant and bar on Wisconsin Avenue, and talk about the lecture.

One week, we made our usual pit stop at the Lehi Grill and discussed the Hodgkin's idea. Moxley's memorable Hodgkin's patient had been a young woman in her twenties, back when he was in training at the Brigham Hospital in Boston. They'd given her different drugs, but none had made a difference. When he met her, she'd been in the women's ward, an open space with partitions between the beds. Eventually, she'd been moved to the one private room on the floor where the sickest patients went to die. He'd watched, helplessly, as the disease painfully consumed her. The similarity in their ages had unnerved him, too. "You realize," he said to me, leaning over his beer, "that this could have happened to you or me."

That night, we began to chew on the idea of combination chemotherapy for Hodgkin's, based on what Frei and Freireich had done on the leukemia ward. We had a general idea and started to sketch it out on bar napkins. People began to look at us in a funny way as our

---

*Jack Moxley left the NCI for Harvard to finish his training. He met the dean at a social event and when asked the same question gave the same answer. He joined the dean as an assistant. Three years later, he became the youngest dean of a medical school in the country at the University of Maryland.

voices rose. It was the combination of excitement and beer, I guess. By the end of the night, we had an idea of what a protocol would look like.

We had one immediate problem: Skipper's data from L1210 mice suggested that you needed four individually effective drugs, given in combination, to have an impact on the cancer. But we didn't really have four drugs that were known to be effective against Hodgkin's. We could use nitrogen mustard or one of its oral variants, chlorambucil or cyclophosphamide. We could use one of the plant alkaloids that had come from the periwinkle plant, vincristine or vinblastine. Everybody thought vinblastine was more effective in treating Hodgkin's disease, but we didn't think the data showed much difference, and vincristine was much less toxic to bone marrow, so we chose vincristine. These were our first two drugs. After more discussion, and another beer, we decided we could add corticosteroids, which suppressed lymphocyte growth in lymph nodes. But we still needed a fourth.

I was reluctant to try BCNU, my explosive pet project, even though I had evidence it worked in advanced Hodgkin's disease. My studies had uncovered a serious problem. The drug caused delayed toxicity, so it was tricky to use.

But there was another drug, ibenzmethyzin, that I thought might be an option. Ibenzmethyzin was a monoamine oxidase (MAO) inhibitor, a chemical that prevents the enzyme, monoamine oxidase, from inactivating monoamine neurotransmitters, increasing their availability to the brain. These neurotransmitters help regulate emotion and maintain neurons, among other things. MAO inhibitors had been developed as antidepressants, without any sense that they might be effective in treating cancer. But it was looking as if this one, at least, was.

It was being tested in Europe in patients with cancer, and I'd heard from Georges Mathé, a visiting French scientist, that there had been some interesting early results in Hodgkin's. Maybe ibenzmethyzin was our fourth drug. Over the next three months, I raced as fast as I could to get patients enrolled in the phase I and II studies of ibenzmethyzin.

It became clear, very quickly, that it worked against Hodgkin's but no other cancer.

Moxley and I now had the four drugs we needed to cobble together a combination chemotherapy regimen. Together, we devised a plan, passing the paper back and forth on the ward when one of us had time to work on it.

Pretty soon, we realized we had another problem. In childhood leukemia, the drug combinations were given intensively, every day, for as long as possible, with the intent to destroy every leukemic cell lingering in the bone marrow and circulating in the bloodstream. Then you stopped and prayed there were enough normal marrow stem cells left to regenerate the bone marrow. Often, there were.

But in patients with solid tumors, we didn't want to damage the marrow. In fact, we needed, as much as possible, to *avoid* damaging it, as our patients would become more fragile if their blood counts dipped. We needed a different dosing schedule, one that killed the Hodgkin's cells but didn't destroy our patients' bone marrow. We had little information to go on, so we decided arbitrarily to give treatment cycles once every twenty-one days.

One day after we had written the protocol, as I was doing the daily "honey bucket" rounds and had my inevitable meet-up in the hallway with Canellos and Moxley, we told Canellos what we were working on and showed him the plan. He laughed. "Don't do something now that's going to embarrass you later in your careers," he said.

Moxley and I took the outline of what we wanted to do and asked Tom Frei if we could meet with him to discuss our ideas. He agreed, and we met in his office on the twelfth floor. Together, Moxley and I explained our process. Frei liked it. But he said it was too early to put ibenzmethyzin, which had now been renamed procarbazine, together with other drugs because there was so little information on long-term side effects. He suggested that we use methotrexate, an anti-leukemia drug used in the VAMP program, in its place.

I was disappointed. But Frei said he'd done a study with methotrexate in lymphomas a few years back. The results weren't impressive, he said, but if you gave it in high enough doses, you got some useful responses. We knew about the study. It had been based on only a handful of patients, and the data weren't very impressive. But we didn't feel we could contradict Frei. We were lucky he was letting us go ahead. He also suggested we use it on a schedule that had been effective in Skipper's mice and in patients with acute leukemia. We weren't sure that a schedule for a mouse would work on a human, but it was the best we had to go on.

With Frei's help, we named the protocol for the drugs we'd chosen. *M* for the *M* in nitrogen mustard, of which cyclophosphamide was a derivative. *O* for Oncovin, the brand name for vincristine (again, we needed a vowel). *M* for methotrexate. And *P* for prednisone, the corticosteroid. MOMP. We settled on a radical ten-week duration for the therapy—four weeks longer than the single-drug chemotherapy that was usually given to treat Hodgkin's. We left Tom's office ready to celebrate. Then all hell broke loose.

We'd neglected to include Paul Carbone in our plans. We should have gone to him first, because he was our immediate boss. But we'd grown accustomed to ignoring him. Jack and I had figured he wouldn't be enthusiastic about our plan—after all, no one was using combination chemotherapy on 12 West—so instinctively we hadn't approached him. We figured he'd have shut us down before we began, and we were right. He wasn't enthusiastic. But we hadn't calculated just how unenthusiastic he'd be, or the depth of his anger because we'd circumvented his authority.

When Frei told Carbone about MOMP, he had a fit. Any study of ours, he complained, would compete for patients with his study, comparing the effectiveness of one drug with another, as part of the research being done with the national clinical cooperative groups— hospitals that were working together on the same trials in order to increase the size of the experiment. Carbone also thought what we had proposed was nuts. There wasn't enough evidence to do this in solid tumors. It would be too dangerous.

And Carbone wasn't the only one we'd ticked off. Ralph Johnson,

the head radiologist, also had a fit when Frei told him about our proposal. He wanted to admit all Hodgkin's patients into his own new
study, using wider fields of radiotherapy. He felt that his study was
much more important than either Carbone's or ours.

Moxley and I had unwittingly found ourselves in our first turf
battle. The bottom line was that Hodgkin's patients were in great de-
mand. And everyone but Frei thought we were proposing something
crazy.

Carbone and Johnson wanted us to forget about it, but Frei stood
behind us. He called a meeting that included Paul Carbone, Ralph
Johnson, Moxley, and me. To our surprise, Freireich also appeared
and pulled up a chair. The meeting quickly became a miniversion of
the Society of Jabbering Idiots, minus the chalkboard.

Johnson, always volatile, immediately launched into a rant. "This
study will be nothing short of malpractice!" he bellowed. "I refuse to
have anything to do with it!"

Moxley and I looked at each other. We refrained from stating
the obvious: we didn't want him to have anything to do with it. Carbone was so angry that his fragmented speech became even more
fractured. Eventually, he trailed off. Freireich sat, uncharacteristically
quiet. He had a smile on his face.

Frei let Moxley and me say our piece, too. Then he offered a solution. We would be allowed to go ahead with MOMP but with certain
limits. We could admit only fourteen patients to the trial so that we
wouldn't hurt anyone else's study much.

Fourteen was a kind of magical number used to determine the
activity of a new drug in a phase II study, which is essentially what our
plans for MOMP were. If you didn't see any promising results in fourteen patients, the odds were you wouldn't, even with more. The drug in
question would then be dropped. But if you saw more than two useful
responses, meaning the tumor had regressed in some individuals, you
could continue.

While Ralph Johnson would solicit early-stage patients for radiotherapy, we would look for those with advanced disease for MOMP,

so that we wouldn't be in competition. We'd have to consult with him on all of our cases. If he thought any of our patients should have radiotherapy, we would have to let him give it to them before we started MOMP.

We'd have to find, admit, and personally care for the fourteen patients ourselves, on top of our regular workload. We wouldn't be able to avail ourselves of the services of any of the other clinical associates, who needed to be available to work on patients in Carbone's study. And we'd have to treat patients in reverse isolation.

That meant no one could enter a patient's room without donning a surgical gown and sterile gloves. It was a precaution. One unique feature of Hodgkin's was that even patients with early-stage disease had an immune defect we could detect with routine skin tests. They were anergic, meaning they were immunologically deficient. This made them susceptible to infections, particularly tuberculosis and fungi but also from bacteria.

There were a lot of patients on 12 West who had something called mycosis fungoides, a skin lymphoma that causes scaly open wounds. These sores were a constant source of infection and a hazard to our patients, whose white blood cell counts could dip very low because of the experimental chemotherapy; we didn't want our Hodgkin's patients exposed to potential infections in the best of circumstances, and particularly not when their bone marrow was taking a beating.

Reverse isolation had been Freireich's idea. "Vince, clean air is better than dirty air," he said, in one of the few times he broke his beatific silence at the meeting. He was working with a new plastic bubble that encircled the beds of leukemic kids. It had special filters that only allowed sterile air to flow in. There kids could survive long periods without infection even when their bone marrow was devoid of normal white blood cells. I was happy to follow his suggestion. By now, I believed most of what Freireich said.

Overall, it was a solution worthy of Solomon. Nobody was totally happy with it, but it allowed everybody to go forward. Frei had gone out on a limb for us; Moxley and I wondered, briefly, if it was worth the trouble we were causing. But after deliberating over a few more beers at Au Pied de Cochon, we decided to forge ahead.

We put our first ad in a medical journal soliciting patients for the study in September 1963. It wasn't easy to find the right ones. We wanted them to be untreated, because prior treatment failure leads cancer cells to smartly avoid the killing effect of a new drug. And patients had to be willing to face the unknown along with us.

We decided early on that we had to be straight with these people. That hadn't always been the case with cancer patients. Memorial Sloan Kettering Cancer Center had once been called Memorial Hospital for Cancer and Allied Diseases. But doctors, even as late as the 1950s and 1960s, often refrained from telling patients their diagnosis. At Sloan Kettering, many patients had been allowed to presume that they had the allied disease.

The Nuremberg Code, established after the experiments performed on Jews imprisoned during World War II, had changed sensibilities about that.[6] The code stated that the voluntary consent of the human subject is absolutely essential. How you got the patient to agree wasn't codified, and there was no one looking over your shoulder to see how you did it. That was left up to the investigator.

Moxley and I met with each patient and explained the disease, what treatments were available, and why we were doing what we were doing. We discussed the risks as well. We told them that it was an experiment, and though we thought it would help, the consequences could be dire, and there was a remote but not inconceivable chance that the treatment could be fatal. And because we knew newly diagnosed cancer patients are too anxious to retain more than about 10 percent of what is said in an initial conversation with their doctors, we held two or three more talks with each person.

A couple of potential patients almost walked away, but finally we had our group. They ranged in age from twenty to fifty. Among them were a twenty-three-year-old woman with a large malignant mass in her chest, who would have opted out but her mother persuaded her to stay; a thirty-five-year-old man from West Virginia with less advanced disease; a forty-four-year-old mother of young children with advanced disease who was afraid to try the program and also afraid not to; and a Peruvian physician.

We also decided to treat Robert Morse—though, because he didn't fit the protocol exactly, he'd be treated "off study," meaning he wouldn't be included in the results. I'd kept him abreast of our plans as Moxley and I developed the rationale. I'd been hesitant about including him. I worried that it would be extra dangerous to someone who'd had prior treatment, because his bone marrow would most likely be depleted. But, as Morse pointed out, he had little to lose. It was possible death versus certain death.

They were all treated as inpatients at the NCI. They would each get three cycles of chemotherapy: cyclophosphamide, vincristine, and methotrexate on day 1, another dose of methotrexate on day 4, another round of cyclophosphamide, vincristine, and methotrexate on day 8, and another dose of methotrexate on day 11. They'd take prednisone, which had no toxic effect on the marrow, daily. We'd wait ten days to let their bone marrow recover before the next cycle would begin. The whole thing would take about two and a half months.

The side effects were almost immediate. The sound of vomiting could be heard along the hallway. Night after night, Moxley and I paced outside the rooms of our patients, fearful of what might happen. Over the weeks that followed, they lost weight and grew listless, and their platelet counts sank lower and lower to dangerous levels.

The methotrexate was very toxic, we realized, at the dose we'd been forced to use to get an effect, especially the last dose on day 11. It compounded the bone marrow suppression caused by the other drugs and caused severe mouth ulcers that provided an entryway for bacteria to get into the bloodstream, putting patients at high risk for infection. We saw foot drop, as a result of the vincristine, though thankfully no one was as deeply affected as the young girl I'd taken care of on Freireich's ward.

But we also saw results, and quickly. Twelve of the fourteen patients went into complete remission—meaning all sign of their tumor was gone. Usually, this happened during the first cycle of chemotherapy, before Johnson had had a chance to give them any radiotherapy. It was a heady day when Moxley walked into one patient's room and said, "It looks like the tumor is taking it on the chin."

Nobody died. But there were some relapses. Using a single drug to treat Hodgkin's, you'd see a tumor go away for a month, maybe two, before it recurred. Of the twelve patients who went into complete remission, nine stayed in remission. Of the three who relapsed, two did so within two months, and one did so at twelve months.

Robert Morse responded well. But he still had evidence of disease when the protocol was completed. His tumor took off then, and he died shortly thereafter. Belatedly, Moxley and I realized that we'd made a mistake in stopping the treatment while it was still working. We'd been too slavish to the protocol and quit simply because that's how we had written the study. It was a lesson I never forgot. But I would see other doctors make the same mistake again and again over the years, including in the case of my friend Lee.

We'd proved it was relatively safe to use this approach in patients with solid tumors. And we'd easily passed the phase II rule and could move on. But it was a jury-rigged study. We had patched it together too quickly to please too many. Ralph Johnson had insisted we give radiotherapy to about a third of the patients, so it was hard to know what effect to attribute to radiation and what to chemotherapy. And we needed a better schedule and a more effective and less toxic drug than methotrexate. With only fourteen patients, and the radiotherapy issue, it was too small a study to draw many conclusions.

We weren't satisfied, but it was a start. We rushed to present our findings at one of the upcoming cancer meetings, that of the American Association for Cancer Research (AACR), which was held in Philadelphia in the spring of 1965. Moxley and I flipped a coin to see who would present at AACR and who would be first author on the eventual paper we would publish. Moxley won the coin toss and elected to be the first author on the paper. He was pleased. "I'm throwing you to the wolves at AACR," he said, laughing. He wasn't kidding.

Every spring, the American Society for Clinical Investigation met in Atlantic City. In the spring of 1964, I'd attended. William Dameshek, a hematologist from the New England Medical Center and the biggest critic of chemotherapy, had formed something he called "the Blood Club." Ostensibly, this smaller group of hematologists gathered to discuss new advances while in town for the larger meeting. Frei and Freireich had been invited, two years in a row to present their work. But it was a setup, an opportunity for others to dress them down. I always wondered why they bothered to go.

By the time I was scheduled to present MOMP at the AACR, I'd already seen Frei and Freireich torn apart in Atlantic City, not to mention the weekly scolding they got at grand rounds. About two hundred people showed up for the session in the City of Brotherly Love, which was being chaired by David Karnofsky, head of the chemotherapy program at Memorial Hospital in New York and a highly regarded expert on leukemia and lymphoma.

In my presentation, I emphasized that in a good number of our patients the tumor had disappeared, according to every test we'd run. This had never been seen before in solid tumors, and I was looking forward to the crowd's reaction. "Our patients were, therefore," I said, savoring the dramatic conclusion, "in complete remission."

Then I waited for the audience's response. Surely there would be many questions about our methodology and the like. But before anyone else could speak, Karnofsky took the microphone. He proceeded to berate me for using the term "complete remission" to describe the disappearance of our patients' tumors.

"That term is reserved for leukemia, where you can actually measure the cells in the bloodstream and bone marrow," he said. "It is not useful in solid tumor chemotherapy."

It seemed to me a silly criticism and one that missed the point of the study. "Complete remission" wasn't used in solid tumor chemotherapy because no one had seen solid tumors completely disappear before. But Karnofsky was a god. I was a nobody.

Karnofsky finally turned over the microphone for questions. I didn't get any shouts about butchery. I didn't get much response at all, in fact. Karnofsky had set the tone. There were a few perfunctory questions about the severity of the side effects. But that was it. Nobody asked about how and why we'd chosen the drugs or the intricate rationale behind the new approach to treatment. The microphone visibly shook in my hand as I thanked Karnofsky for moderating the panel.

I'd officially joined the ranks of the likes of Louie the Hawk and Frei and Freireich. I was a chemotherapist. And I'd gotten a pretty good taste of what it was like to act counter to the conventional wisdom. I returned home, more determined than ever to earn the right to the phrase "complete remission." There was only one way to do it: my patients needed not only to respond but to survive. We needed a bigger study, and a better one.

4

MOPP

I knew why other doctors were reluctant to follow our lead. Cancer was among the most challenging of diseases. We knew almost nothing about why it happened or how it happened, and thus a sense of powerlessness surrounded it, even among scientists.

And medicine is, by definition, a conservative field. It should be, in a way. People's lives depend upon it. But here was the problem with cancer: none of the other treatments were working. If we didn't push, people who wanted to live died.

Most of the studies presented at AACR were lab based and boring. The tools available to study cancer at the cellular level were limited. It was the proverbial black box. You could examine it but couldn't pry the lid off and look inside. The clinical studies were even more limited. Most were reports on the use of new derivatives of old drugs or studies of the pharmacology of old drugs. Pharmacology in those days was the basic science of the cancer field. I was struck by the sense of futility pervading the meeting.

What Karnofsky didn't know, when he was dressing me down at the AACR, was that he hadn't cowed me into submission. I'd continued to do work on procarbazine, the drug that Frei had encouraged us to dump in favor of methotrexate, when we were creating MOMP, because he said we didn't know enough about its toxicity. I now knew not only that it was more effective against lymphoma than methotrexate but that it was less toxic to the bone marrow.

By the time I was presenting MOMP, I had already begun recruiting for the next study, an improved MOMP. In this one, I would substitute procarbazine for methotrexate, which meant we needed a new acronym. MOMP would become MOPP.

The dosing and scheduling of the drugs in MOPP would be different, too. Frei had urged us to use MOMP on a schedule based on how VAMP was given, which meant relying on an assumption that the rate of growth for Hodgkin's cells was the same as that for leukemia. I wasn't so sure that was true, but it was all we had to go on.

Shortly thereafter, though, a new research tool had become available: tritiated thymidine, a radioactive hydrogen atom capable of attaching itself to thymidine, one of the four chemical components of DNA. If you dosed cells with it as they were going through DNA synthesis, in preparation for replicating, a small subset of cells integrated it into their DNA. It became like a cellular GPS, a tracking device.

To follow the activity of the treated cells, you took a slide smeared with the cells and overlaid it with photographic film. Under a microscope, the radioactive particles embedded in the cells exposed the film, appearing as black-silver dots over cells that had taken it up. In this way, we could closely follow the cells' behavior.

Cancer cells are most vulnerable to chemotherapy when they're dividing, so the rate of cell division mattered. I wanted to know how often leukemia cells divided, and in comparison with Hodgkin's cells. I corralled Ron Yankee, who worked in a nearby lab at the NCI and who'd been my senior resident at the University of Michigan, to help me.

Yankee and I gave repeated pulses of tritiated thymidine over a twelve-hour period to our trial mice, injecting the chemical directly into their bellies, which were distended with cancer cells we'd implanted there. After the duration of a full cell cycle (about twelve hours), we'd extract cells from their bellies and, with Howard Skipper often standing over our shoulders, slide a sample under the microscope and count how many cells had gone through cell division during a single cycle.

Skipper thought we were wasting our time and that the cell-counting studies he'd done in L1210 mice were all we needed to devise a dosing schedule. But I wanted to be sure.

It was tedious work involving hours of looking down the barrel of a microscope counting dotted cells as they marched through the phases of cell division. But it was worth it. The percentage of a tumor that goes through cell division is called the growth fraction. As we watched, we observed an amazing fact. Every single leukemic cell in L1210 went through cell division every twelve hours. The growth fraction was 100 percent.

This was a startling observation. If cells are most vulnerable to the drugs used in chemotherapy during cell division, the L1210 cells were supremely vulnerable, because they all went through cell division in every cycle. But was that true of other cancers, like Hodgkin's?

I wanted to study human Hodgkin's cells, but that was impossible. There were too few to work with, and we couldn't repeatedly take tissue samples from the tumors of humans without causing distress to the humans in question. But Mortimer Mendelsohn, a scientist at the University of Pennsylvania, had done a study on the growth fraction of solid tumors, a category that included Hodgkin's, in rodents. His research suggested that the growth fraction of cells in solid tumors didn't exceed 20 percent at any given time.

That meant a lot of cells in solid tumors wouldn't be dividing over the time frame of a single cycle. And if that were true, we'd need to give treatment for long periods, much longer than the schedule used for VAMP. It would probably take many months, in fact, to catch all the cancerous cells when it became their turn to divide. That was a potential problem; we needed to spare the normal bone marrow. And for that, we had to understand how cell turnover in the bone marrow worked. Seymour Perry, a hematologist studying bone marrow growth, had looked at the growth rate of cells in normal human marrow using tritiated thymidine. Yankee and I now did the same work in mice and found that it took mouse marrow cells half the time to complete their life cycle that it took human marrow cells.

We then did the lab work exposing both normal human and mouse marrow to a high dose of chemotherapy and compared the recovery times. It turned out that in mice everything took half as long as it did in humans. All our dosing schedules, thus far, had been based on the L1210 mice. This didn't matter so much in Frei and Freireich's clinical studies in leukemia, because they needed to blast away the marrow cells. But because we didn't want to damage marrow this time around if we could help it, it was important to know that mouse and human marrow behaved differently. We now understood that we couldn't use the schedule developed as tolerable in mice directly in humans, which is how we had given methotrexate in MOMP. We would have to develop schedules around the recovery time of normal human marrow and treat for a long time, to catch all the malignant cells when they were dividing.

The studies we did with tritiated thymidine in the marrow of mice and men and in leukemias and solid tumors were the first of their kind and proved immensely useful in the design of the MOPP protocol. From these data, we deduced the sequence of events bone marrow went through from damage to recovery.

In a human, if you shut down the bone marrow factory with a big dose of a toxic chemical, the marrow is left with a reserve of white blood cells and platelets. The reserve has an ample enough supply to last for about a week to ten days. If you did a blood count during this time, the cell count would appear normal, even though the stem cell factory (stem cells generate all the cells in the marrow) had been shut down. But the damage had been done, and the storage compartment would be emptying.

However, a second dose of a drug that is toxic to the marrow during the first ten days isn't as damaging as the first. There are two reasons for this. The more mature cells left in the storage compartment aren't all that sensitive to chemotherapy in the first place. And the stem cells would have been rendered quiescent by the first dose. Cells that are going through a lot of cell division, as stem cells normally do, are most vulnerable to the toxic effects of chemotherapy. Inactive cells, however, aren't dividing, so they're less susceptible to damage.

From day 9 after a dose of chemotherapy until about day 18, patients are out of white blood cells and platelets. While the stem cells in the marrow are awakening, they are not making many cells. This is the period of greatest danger for acquiring an infection or bleeding. After day 18, the marrow wakes up again in earnest, and the stem cells begin furiously churning out more white blood cells and platelets, although few of them leave the marrow until the storage compartment is full again. If you give another big dose of drug between days 14 and 18, it will cause severe marrow toxicity that could be fatal to the freshly dividing cells.

By day 21, the storage compartment is full again, and signs of recovery—in the form of brand-new white blood cells and platelets circulating in the bloodstream—are in evidence. From day 21 to day 28, blood counts returns to normal.

Based on what we'd learned, we decided to give MOPP in two-week cycles. Patients would get two full doses of nitrogen mustard and two full doses of vincristine by IV on days 1 and 8. Procarbazine and prednisone, neither of which was particularly toxic to the bone marrow, would both be given once daily, by mouth, for fourteen days. The patient would then rest for two weeks. The next cycle would start on day 28. This schedule, we thought, while intense, would get us around damaging the bone marrow too much.

We knew that solid tumors had a low growth fraction, so MOPP had to be given safely for a long time to get rid of Hodgkin's. We needed to get the drugs in on as tight a schedule as possible to be sure we maximized the killing effect on the tumors. The question was, how many cycles to use? We knew ten weeks of treatment with MOMP, even though it was a month longer than the standard duration for single-drug treatment, hadn't been enough. Too many patients, including Robert Morse, still had tumor—and had still been responding— when we stopped.

If the growth fraction of Hodgkin's cells was, like other solid tumors, around 20 percent, then we would need at least five tightly packed cycles. Because we were guessing here, we settled on six cycles.

In homage to Morse, Moxley and I had created a novel rule. We'd never stop treatment as long as a patient was still responding to the therapy. Our patients would get as many cycles as they needed to go into complete remission, and two more after that. Even if patients went into remission after only two or three cycles, they'd get a minimum of six. We knew we'd get flack for sure. No one had ever tried using combinations of toxic drugs in cancer patients for the ten weeks we'd treated with MOMP, much less the six months we were proposing now. But it seemed rational to us.

We also knew, from MOMP, that patients' reactions to drugs would differ, depending on their health. Sicker patients, in general, could tolerate less chemotherapy, although they needed it more. One factor that would screw up the sequence of events in bone marrow recovery was earlier exposure to chemotherapy or radiotherapy. Prior treatment meant the stem cell compartment was already damaged, so the compartment was quicker to disappear and slower to come back. Because of this, we needed to do the study on previously untreated patients to see how well our rationale for sparing bone marrow worked.

If our assumptions were correct, we had to stay on schedule so that the tumor didn't have time to grow back. We wanted to keep clobbering it until it was gone. And Skipper's data indicated that it was of paramount importance to expose the cancer cells to all four drugs at the same time so that the cells would not become drug resistant. We anticipated that some patients' blood counts might not return to normal by day 28. If that happened, we'd go ahead with treatment on schedule, but we'd sacrifice some fraction of the doses of each drug, using a sliding scale for dose reduction. It was better to use some portion of each drug than to skip a dose or change the schedule.

Finally, we decided to jettison a mainstay of single-drug treatment—maintenance therapy. In studies like Carbone's, which focused on a single drug, patients who responded were "maintained" on treatment. That is, after achieving a good partial response, chemotherapy was continued for as long as the tumor didn't grow back. This practice was rapidly becoming de rigueur. The trouble was, when you compared the survival rates of patients on maintenance chemotherapy with those whose treatment was stopped and restarted when the tumor grew back, there wasn't any difference. Eventually, they died.

Our intent for MOPP was to put patients into complete remission, stop treatment, and observe them. This was the only way you could tell if you had cured the patient, and we wanted that as our end point.

Carbone didn't like this at all.

"What you're proposing is unethical," he said. "Maintenance therapy prolongs the duration of responses." We were standing in the patient corridor on 12 West, trying to keep our voices down so that the patients didn't hear.

"But there's no evidence that maintenance treatment actually keeps people alive longer," I shot back. "If patients are cured, they don't need further chemotherapy. And we need to know if we cured them. And if they aren't cured, it won't make a difference in survival if we restart treatment later."

"If I were you," Carbone said, "I'd be careful about the way you're throwing the word 'cure' around." He walked off in a huff.

With Frei's support, we'd be able to go ahead, but things were getting nasty with Carbone.

We started recruiting patients for MOPP in early 1964, putting ads in medical journals, at medical meetings, and the like, indicating that we needed patients with advanced disease who had received no prior treatment. In most centers, you had to take what came in the door. And what tended to come in the door, with Hodgkin's, were desperately ill patients with advanced disease who had been treated with the chemotherapy of the day, usually chlorambucil, and were now out of options. Either their insurance had run out, or they were facing certain death, and they wanted another shot at something.

They would not be candidates for MOPP. We needed newly diagnosed patients with advanced disease to see how the regimen truly worked. If we were successful, we could then try it on previously treated patients. We already knew we wouldn't be getting many patients from the Washington, D.C., area. The local doctors were hostile to the NIH. We were government funded and provided care free of charge. They thought we were unfair competition.

The problem with patients who came from afar was that they needed a place to stay. This would be a bigger study than MOMP. We couldn't house them all in the hospital. Frei and Freireich had already run into this problem and solved it by persuading Gordon Zubrod, who ran the department, to make an arrangement for the NCI to virtually buy a motel in downtown Bethesda, the Town and Country Inn, to house patients and their families, at no cost. It was located on Rockville Pike, walking distance from the NIH. We'd gotten permission to use the facilities for our MOPP patients and their families now, too, so we could accept people from anywhere in the United States.

Initially, the patients trickled in very slowly. The first was a forty-eight-year-old woman with massive signs of tumor in her chest. The next two were both young men in their twenties. We treated them with MOPP, and all three went into complete remission. Because we were treating for an unheard-of six months, we didn't want to take on any more patients until these three had completed their course of treatment. So far, though, things were looking good.

Meanwhile, Zubrod had put together task forces on the various subtypes of cancer, the members of which came from different hospitals and universities, to see if together they could accelerate progress.

He'd made Tom Frei chair of the lymphoma task force; their first meeting was held at the NCI in the spring of 1964, after we'd started MOMP. Frei asked me to make an informal presentation about our current work and to outline the MOPP protocol.

We met in a large room with a long oval table at which about twenty luminaries, mostly professors of hematology, sat elbow to elbow. Frei said he wanted to go around the table and have each person discuss what he was doing at his institution. He started with the person on my left and went around the table the other way, so I would be last. By the time he'd gone halfway around the table, it was obvious that no one was doing anything new, and survival rates weren't changing. There was no plan, no hypothesis, under test. One ho-hum drug was being compared with another.

When he got to me, he said, "Vince, why don't you go to the blackboard and tell the group what you're doing." I rose, a bit shakily, and took up the chalk. This was nothing like the Society of Jabbering Idiots. The room was silent as I wrote on the board, the tap and squeak of the chalk audible to all. When I was done, I turned to face my colleagues. They were clearly shocked, especially when I said it was the intent of the MOPP study to try to cure Hodgkin's. Wayne Rundles, a famous professor from Duke and the developer of chlorambucil, one of the most popular drugs used to treat Hodgkin's, had visibly winced. Then he raised his hand. "Dr. DeVita," he said, "do your patients *speak* to you after you do this to them?"

I knew exactly what he was getting at. He didn't believe a cure was possible, and he thought we were putting patients through hell for nothing. Frei spared me having to tussle with Rundles by changing the subject. But Frei's message to the group—delivered via me—was clear: *You guys aren't doing anything new.* Their message, in return, had been equally clear: *You guys are nuts.*

Things looked great, on the one hand. But the ground was starting to shake under my feet. R. Lee Clark, a cancer surgeon and the president and founder of the MD Anderson Cancer Center in Houston, Texas, one of the three freestanding cancer centers in the country at that time, was putting pressure on Frei to build a chemotherapy program there. MD Anderson didn't have one, and Clark, sensing that the field was growing, wanted to ensure that his center remained cutting-edge.

Rumor had it that Clark had been leaning on Frei for some time and Frei had been putting him off. Now the word was that Clark was calling Frei every month to tell him how much money he'd already lost by not going there. This had to hurt. Clark could pay a salary at least five times what Frei was making in his government job. Tom had four kids of his own and was supporting the children of his late brother-in-law as well. I didn't see how he could hold out much longer.

This would be bad news for me. I'd learned that in order to do anything outside the mores of medicine, you needed someone in a high place, or at least high enough, to run interference. Zubrod did it for Frei and Freireich. Having spent the better part of a year on the wards watching Freireich's behavior, I now referred to Zubrod as "the great umbrella." It was clear to me that he used his power and prestige to protect the more adventurous members of his staff.

Frei, in turn, had been an umbrella for me; without him, I wasn't sure if I'd be able to continue with MOPP. I also didn't know what would happen to Freireich. He was as volatile and outrageous as ever. Without Frei to smooth the feathers he ruffled, I didn't see how he could stay. I was betting Frei would take Freireich with him if he went.

Our MOPP trial, though small, was going well. But before I knew it, my two-year period as a clinical associate was nearing an end. It was decision time. George Canellos was going back to Massachusetts General Hospital and then to Hammersmith Hospital for more training under the great British hematologist Sir John Dacie. Jack Moxley wanted to go back to Peter Bent Brigham Hospital in Boston. They were like lemmings going home.

There was nothing for me back at GW. And I was still insecure about my academic credentials. So I applied for a two-year residency at two big-time medical programs, Duke and Yale. Duke was home to Eugene Stead; Paul Beeson was at Yale. Both were legends, regarded as worthy successors to the great Sir William Osler, the father of internal medicine and one of the four co-founders of the Johns Hopkins School of Medicine.

I was accepted into both programs. Each indicated that I didn't need conventional training, given what I'd learned at the NCI, and proposed that my course of study would deviate from the traditional plan. In the end, I chose Yale. For the first six months of the first year, I'd be a conventional resident at Yale–New Haven Hospital, and for the remainder of the year I'd be chief resident at Yale's VA hospital. I'd spend the next year as a hematology fellow with the chief of hematology, Stuart Finch.

Rall wasn't happy. He wanted me to stay at the NCI. As an incentive, he said he'd keep me on its payroll while I was away. It was fantastic news. A senior resident at Yale made about $4,000 a year. I was making $11,000 in the Public Health Service at the rank of lieutenant commander. I quickly accepted the offer.

In April 1965, four months before my stint as a clinical associate was up, Frei left for MD Anderson. As I feared, he took Freireich with him. I managed to recruit and treat five more MOPP patients before I left for Yale in July. Paul Carbone promised he'd see that patients were accrued to the MOPP study while I was gone. I wasn't sure I could trust him, so I asked Arthur Serpick, who headed the lymphoma program at our Baltimore center, to enlist patients for MOPP, too. I enticed him with the promise that he'd be a co-author on any paper that came out of it.

I liked the fact that I was now going to an elite program and that the NCI was paying me to come back, but I was worried about MOPP. Two years seemed like a long time to be away from it.

At Yale, I quickly realized that I was way ahead of my peers. I was already an independent physician with a good deal of experience. In some ways, I had more experience than my attendings, who were technically my superiors.

But technicalities mattered. You could tell where people stood in the pecking order at a glance. Resident physicians wore white pants

and short white coats. Senior doctors wore long white coats over normal attire. If there was a difference of opinion, the ones wearing the
long white coats won automatically.

I was technically only a resident, but I often had a better idea of
how to treat patients with leukemia or lymphomas than the senior
doctors, given what I'd just seen at the NCI.

I regularly encountered patients with pseudomonas aeruginosa
and pseudomonas rectal infections and easily picked up on them. I
knew, because Freireich had taught me, that in people with good
white blood cell counts, pseudomonas aeruginosa usually causes a
pus-filled abscess in the rectum that you can feel, but that leukemic
patients have too few functioning white cells to cluster together and
form one. At the NCI, I'd learned to recognize the condition in these
patients by checking if the rectal area was tender to the touch. In
the presence of a high fever, that was all I needed to know to quickly
start treating a patient with high-powered combinations of intravenous antibiotics. It was life or death.

It was the same with pseudomonas meningitis, which I'd learned—
from Freireich—to treat by injecting the antibiotic polymyxin B
directly into the spinal fluid, despite what it said on the vial. But I
couldn't convince the chief of infectious diseases at Yale that the
patients had these infections, or how to treat them. And in the home
of Professor Paul Beeson, who had written about the dangers of using
antibiotics in combination, you just didn't do this kind of thing. As a
result, I watched leukemic patients die.

They also often developed lobar pneumonia, pneumonia that
affects a large area of the lung, which was generally believed to be
caused by bacteria, klebsiella or pneumococcus. But at the NCI, we
had discovered that in leukemia patients a fungus named *Aspergillus
fumigatus* caused the condition and resulted in what looked like an
ordinary pneumonia. The tendency was to treat it with antibiotics.
The problem, of course, was that a fungus does not respond to ordinary antibiotics. This one in particular had to be treated with a
difficult-to-use antifungal medication that Freireich had also taught

me how to administer. When I saw the condition in patients with leukemia and pointed it out to the chief of infectious diseases at Yale, he didn't believe me—even when the lab tests proved my point. He insisted that the fungus had to be a contaminant, something that had been introduced to the specimen by accident. Treating leukemic patients with an antifungal was simply not the practice at the time. The patients weren't treated with the right medication, and many succumbed to the fungal infections.*

Patients on chemotherapy were bleeding to death for lack of platelets. I tried to get platelets for transfusions, but my boss, the big boss of hematology, Stuart Finch, under whom I'd be doing my second year at Yale, said there was no evidence that they worked. Nat Berlin, the NCI's clinical director, a well-known hematologist and the one who'd threatened to fire Freireich for using them, had told him so, he said. Ergo, at Yale, I watched patients bleed to death.

Things came to a head one day when I had to present a patient with advanced Hodgkin's disease to Stuart Finch. When I was done, Finch leaned over in a conspiratorial manner and said, "Don't send him to Calabresi, he might give him that combination chemotherapy stuff."

Paul Calabresi was the head of the clinical pharmacology section at Yale, which had been established to test cancer drugs coming from the pharmacology lab. It was the same department where nitrogen mustard was first tested and was really the first section of medical oncology in the country. Calabresi was a pioneer. He had been at the meeting where Frei had asked me to present my data on MOMP and MOPP. He was one of the few who had—quietly—let me know he was excited by them.

But the Yale staff was frightened of chemotherapy. They felt it did harm to the patients; they didn't even want to rotate on Calabresi's

---

*He was actually a very good doctor. I learned a lot from him. And our sparring over the use of antifungals led him to become interested in aspergillosis. He went on to become one of the country's leading experts in the disease.

service. Finch had no idea that I was the guy who had developed combination chemotherapy for Hodgkin's at the NCI. He told me to palliate the patient—lessen the symptoms but not try to cure the disease—with the same old drug, chlorambucil.

The only bright spot was Beeson. It was true he was the source of the treat-with-one-antibiotic-at-a-time protocol. But that was a rule being used by others out of the context in which he'd created it. In my direct experience with the man, he had a fine and flexible mind, and it was exciting to watch him work. We had what were called "professor's rounds" each week, where we presented a few tough cases to Beeson for his advice. Because Beeson was a well-known infectious disease expert, we always looked around for a case to stump him.

One week, I was really excited because I had found a great case for him. One of my patients was a middle-aged black woman with a fever of undetermined origin, or FUO, as we often shortened the term. We thought she had an infection, but we couldn't figure out what it was. We cultured her blood, looking for signs of endocarditis, an inflammation of the inner layer of the heart due to infection. Nothing. We cultured her urine, looking for a kidney infection. Nada. We did every other test we could think of and had not found any infectious source for the fever. I'd found nothing of note on the physical examination, either. She was a complete puzzle.

At rounds with Beeson, I stood straight in my white starched jacket and pants and presented the case, proud of my recall of all the minute details of her history. He listened politely as he stood amid our bevy of residents and interns, all in starched white suits, fanned out by the bedside. Beeson was always unfailingly polite.

When I finished, he walked to the edge of the patient's bed. "Do you have headaches?" he asked her. "Yes," she said. I was instantly mortified. I hadn't thought to ask her that. The woman had a big Afro, a common style at the time. Beeson reached over and slipped his hand under her Afro and ran his hand along her temple. She winced as his fingers ran over the speed bump of her inflamed temporal artery, instead of the flat surface that should have been there.

He turned to me. "She has temporal arteritis. Do you have another case?" And then he walked out of the room.

Temporal arteritis is an inflammatory disease of blood vessels. Although not an infectious disease, it does cause fever (and headaches) and needs to be considered in the differential diagnosis, the process by which doctors narrow down to a diagnosis. To do this you start by making a list of all the likely diagnoses, putting the most likely on top, and work your way through the possibilities. Temporal arteritis had not even made my list. Because a branch of the temporal artery feeds the back of the eyeball and blockage can cause blindness, missing the diagnosis could have had serious consequences for this woman.

And I'd missed it.

I'd been looking for typical causes of fever in a woman her age. I hadn't asked her about headaches. And her bushy hair had deterred me from examining her scalp. I felt as if I had been demoted to medical student. That day at lunch in the cafeteria, I slid next to Beeson at a table and apologized for missing the diagnosis. "How were you able to make the diagnosis so quickly?" I asked.

He looked me in the eye. "Vince, everyone knows I'm a specialist in infectious diseases. By the time I get to see a patient, they've ruled out all the obvious causes of fever. So I often start at the bottom of the list, looking for the thing most likely to have been overlooked. I took one look at her hair and guessed that no one had looked under it. And I was right. A new pair of eyes often sees something obvious that the primary doctor, staring at the chart and the patient every day, has missed."

I had learned to recognize the people I could learn from, and Beeson was one of them. He was the sole reason I wanted to be there. But in January, there was another blow. Paul Beeson announced that he was going to England to be the Nuffield Professor of Medicine at Oxford, the chair that had been occupied by Sir William Osler. I was stunned. Beeson was the reason I'd come to Yale. And given my experience so far, he was the only reason I was staying.

Before Beeson left, I asked to have lunch with him. We sat at a round table in the Yale hospital cafeteria. As people milled around us,

I shared my feelings. *Hell, what do I have to lose?* I thought. Beeson was going anyhow. I told him about Freireich and the NIH and what I'd seen there and the difficulties I was having persuading people at Yale to be more heroic. Beeson listened quietly.

When I was done, he nodded and said, "Vince, let me tell you a story." Some years earlier, he said, he'd gone to India and had been asked to make rounds on a ward devoted to patients afflicted with typhoid fever, a bacterial illness transmitted by contaminated food and water. It's rare in the United States but common in tropical and subtropical areas.

"The Indian resident presented about twenty-five cases of typhoid fever to me that morning," said Beeson. "The first two he described as 'typical.' The next twenty or so he described as 'atypical.' 'Why are you calling so many cases atypical when they're the majority?' I asked him. And he said, 'Because, Professor Beeson, that's the way you described typical cases in your book.'"

At the time, Beeson was the co-editor of the most famous textbook of medicine and a specialist in infectious diseases. Beeson said, "I told him, 'I've only seen three cases of typhoid fever, personally, before today.'" The Indian resident would not believe what his eyes were seeing because of something written by a great professor who had less experience in his lifetime than the Indian resident had in a day.

"Listen and learn from what you have seen with your own eyes," said Beeson. "They are probably correct." As I sat there with the great professor, my short white coat had not mattered at all. He had repudiated his own staff in favor of the observations of a lowly resident. And he'd taught me something important about trusting my instincts. That lunch had made the months of difficulties worth it. Almost.

Not long after that, Beeson's replacement, Phil Bondy, came on board. He sided with Finch with regard to chemotherapy. He didn't want it on his wards. Calabresi was ousted and replaced by a guy who was nice but mostly a lab jock who preferred testing drugs in mice.

In July, exactly a year after I'd started at Yale, I got a call from Dave Rall saying he could use me back at the NIH if I'd be willing to dump the hematology fellowship. Without Beeson, there was no reason for me to stay at Yale, so I agreed. Besides, by now I had come to believe both Stead's and Beeson's original assessment: I didn't really need that extra training.

The NCI had undergone some reorganization since Frei and Freireich had left. The chemotherapy division was still led, overall, by Gordon Zubrod; Sy Perry, a hematologist from the University of Southern California, had taken Tom Frei's job as chief of the medicine branch. No one had yet replaced Jay Freireich—not that anyone ever could.

Neither Paul Carbone nor the guy he had assigned to the MOPP study had treated any patients with that drug protocol while I was away. Art Serpick had treated six cases at the Baltimore center, and the early results looked pretty good. But we needed more patients. It took me six months to get the study on track. By early 1967, we had treated thirty patients with MOPP, all of whom had been admitted with very advanced, symptomatic disease. In 90 percent of cases, all their tumor disappeared.

I presented the preliminary results at the AACR meeting in May 1967. The authors on that abstract were, as promised, V. T. DeVita and A. Serpick.[1]

The results were remarkably different from what anyone had seen before in Hodgkin's disease. But the Karnofsky experience was still fresh in my mind. I wanted to wait to publish the paper so we could present the four-year disease-free survival curves, the hallmark of a cure. No one had ever done that before.

By 1969, we'd accrued forty-three patients and decided that we'd publish the results of that group of patients. I submitted another abstract to the AACR meeting, in the spring of 1969, as a progress report.[2]

By now, Paul Carbone was chief of medicine, and I'd taken his job as head of the solid tumor service. He had sign-off rights on all papers coming from the branch. To my irritation, given how much flack he'd given me for MOMP and MOPP, he put his name on the abstract. It was now V. T. DeVita, A. Serpick, and P. P. Carbone.

Carbone's tendency to add his name to papers wasn't unknown. George Canellos, who'd come back to the NCI as a senior investigator and was as acerbic as ever, had noted the "and" that often preceded Carbone's name and dubbed him "Andy." The moniker stuck. So many people heard us refer to him that way, though not to his face, that some thought it was actually his name and used it when addressing him. "That's not my name," he'd answer irritably.*

It was galling to have to add his name to the study. The authorship on the abstract would carry over to the authorship on the paper we'd eventually publish in a journal. When I mentioned adding Tom Frei's and Jack Moxley's names as authors, Carbone said he didn't think they merited it. Neither had stayed involved. Never mind that Moxley had helped create the idea in the first place and that Frei had cleared the way for us. But it was a battle I couldn't win by myself.

I personally followed every patient on the MOPP study, including those in Baltimore, although Art Serpick cared for those patients on a daily basis. I logged all the details of each patient on a big chart that I rolled up in a scroll and carried with me. The clinical associates got a kick out of seeing me walk the halls with my "Dead Sea Scrolls."

Given my experience with Karnofsky, I knew that when we published the results, we'd face questions about how we could be sure that all the tumor was gone. So we developed a novel and strict protocol for assessing the presence or absence of tumor at the end of treatment: every test that was abnormal at diagnosis had to be normal for us to call a response a complete remission. If there were any residual abnormalities, we did repeat biopsies.

We used a technique called lymphangiogram to check how clear the lymph nodes were. We'd inject dye-stained radiopaque contrast

---

*Although the stories I recount about Paul Carbone are factual, I believe they *were* a reflection of the hostile environment at the time. He, in reality, was a caring, talented physician-scientist. After I was appointed over him as director of the Division of Cancer Treatment, he left the NCI and became director of Wisconsin's Comprehensive Cancer Center, where he united a once disparate center. He was so well regarded there that when he died unexpectedly at age seventy, the center was named after him.

material into lymph channels between a patient's toes. We could follow the progress of the blue dye up the foot until it disappeared in the lymph channels, which went deeper into the legs and then the abdomen. Then we'd take an ordinary X-ray of the abdomen. The contrast material stayed in the lymph nodes for as long as a year, enabling us to visualize lymph nodes we couldn't otherwise see and feel while minimizing the patient's discomfort. Our patients used to joke about their purple feet.

We'd done a lymphangiogram on each patient every year for at least four years, giving us five years during which we could visualize their abdominal nodes. We quickly found out that if a patient with advanced disease remained in a complete remission with no further therapy for four years, he or she rarely relapsed. The patient was cured.

Hodgkin's disease is divided into four stages, denoted by the roman numerals I through IV. The higher the number, the more advanced the cancer. Each stage is also classified as A or B: A means the patient is asymptomatic; B means the person has symptoms of the disease. The B cases are the worst. Eighty-eight percent of our patients were stage IVB—as bad as it gets.

One man was as sick as I have ever seen anyone with Hodgkin's. He had stage IVB. He'd been spiking high fevers, lost thirty pounds, and had tumor everywhere, including his liver. He was in such rough shape that I didn't expect him to live through the treatment. But he went into remission within two cycles of MOPP—every bit of tumor gone. We thought it was a bit of a miracle; he thought it was a miracle, too. But this kind of thing was happening over and over again.

Unlike with MOMP, we were treating these patients as outpatients. That meant they would come to the NCI and get their therapy and either go home, if they lived close by, or stay in the nearby Town and Country Inn. Patients would show up at the appointed time and head for the chemo room, where the nurses would install their IVs and start the drip. Patients complained of a metallic taste that hit the backs of their mouths the second the nitrogen mustard entered their veins. The nurses took to keeping a jar of peppermint candy next to the door. It became standard procedure for patients to grab one and pop it in their mouths before starting the drip.

The nausea set in about forty-five minutes after the IV had been removed. Then the patients would vomit every few minutes for the next eight hours. We had arranged for a shuttle bus to take patients to and from the hotel. But few patients used the bus. The nausea often got the better of them before they could make it to the curb. Instead, they took to walking in a diagonal line that went from the clinical center, across the lawn of the National Library of Medicine and the highway that bordered the NIH campus, and back to their hotel. One patient told me he always saved the barf bag from the plane he'd taken on the way down specifically for the walk back to the hotel. "The people driving along the road and the other pedestrians probably think I'm the local drunk, or worse," he said, not without humor.

Eventually, the path became so worn that it formed a grassless rift in the lawn, a ragged track that the patients dubbed "the Chemo Trail." Some years later, the grounds people would give up trying to reseed the grass and paved the path to make a walkway. The patients who happened to be in town when this happened carved their initials in the wet concrete.

In time, after patients had done a few rounds of MOPP, they didn't even need to get the nitrogen mustard to start vomiting. They'd see me walk into the room or hear the sound of an IV pole rattling as it was being wheeled down the hallway to the chemo room, and, like Pavlov's stimulus-trained dogs, they'd throw up.

At the hotel, despite their nausea, they were comfortable, because almost everyone there was a cancer patient. Wheelchairs and IVs were de rigueur among the clientele, who ran the gamut of professions, from grocers to CEOs.

The IVB patients were willing to put up with anything. They knew how sick they were. And because they were so symptomatic already, they often immediately felt better with MOPP, as their tumors melted away. That went a long way toward compensating for the side effects. As one patient bluntly put it, "What's my other choice? Death."

But he wasn't despairing when he said it. Sick and frightened as they were, these patients knew they were pioneers.

It was tougher dealing with the patients who were IIIA, because they might be symptom-free when they joined our study, even if they had tumor in their lymph nodes. They often went from feeling fine to wretchedly ill in one cycle. The protocol made you sick as a dog, and they felt as if the drugs were making them ill rather than destroying their tumor. Because of this, it was sometimes hard to convince them that the treatment was necessary to save their lives.

One patient, the eighteen-year-old son of the secretary of housing and urban development, was stage IIIA and felt fine when he was admitted. His case had been diagnosed early, when a routine X-ray picked up signs of a tumor. It was a lucky catch, and he should have been an easy cure. But after one round of MOPP, he refused to continue and discharged himself. He thought we were just making him sicker.

His reasoning wasn't totally irrational. We weren't sure we were curing anybody long-term at that point. But we were optimistic. And the alternatives weren't good. He died within a couple of years.

Four years after getting dressed down in public by Karnofsky for using the term "complete remission," I went back to the AACR to present our most recent findings. The complete remission rate for MOPP, over four years, was 80 percent—the highest ever reported. And we had relapse-free survival curves that were flattening out at two years, meaning the rate of relapse was declining with time, another hallmark of a curative treatment.[3]

When I finished my talk, the chair of the session, Charlie Huguley, interceded before the questions could start. Charlie was a well-known hematologist and chairman of the Southeastern Cancer Study Group, a large cooperative clinical trials group made up of a dozen institutions. This time the comment was positive. Huguley had a lot of experience with Hodgkin's and knew that what I was presenting was radically different from anything seen before, and he said so. The response from the audience was equally gratifying. No one questioned the use of the term "complete remission."

A year later, in 1970, we published the paper describing the MOPP results in the first forty-three patients in the *Annals of Internal Medicine*. It became the most cited paper in the history of the publication.[4]

Considering what a radical departure MOPP was from traditional treatment, I got a surprisingly positive response from within the medical field. For the first time, chemotherapists actually had a treatment to prescribe that might cure their patients.

In 1974, chemotherapy—now known as medical oncology—was established as an official subspecialty of medicine, complete with its own board exams. MOPP had helped make that happen. It was heady. A field that had been widely derided as dangerous quackery had become not just reputable but an accepted new avenue of treatment.

But not everyone was thrilled. Some took a wait-and-see approach or were openly skeptical and refused to try MOPP on patients. And in fact, some physicians remained downright hostile. The worst response came from radiotherapists. Until now, they'd had a free hand with lymphoma and Hodgkin's patients at every stage of disease, only passing them on to chemotherapists or internists when all else failed.

Now almost all patients with advanced disease were being treated with MOPP. And because most were being cured, there was no need to use radiation to alleviate the symptoms of the disease.

Meanwhile, Skipper's inverse rule nagged at us. It wasn't long before we decided it would be smart to test MOPP against radiotherapy for early-stage Hodgkin's disease. If MOPP cured patients with lots of tumor, we reasoned, shouldn't it work even better in early-stage patients? The answer was yes. Twice as many patients in our study stayed free of disease after MOPP as after radiation therapy alone.

It was a startling result, so surprising that most radiotherapists refused to believe it. Their concession was to give MOPP along with radiotherapy. Radiotherapists began to lose referrals as the management of the disease shifted to medical oncologists. As a result, many began to refuse to cooperate in large studies of early-stage patients unless radiotherapy was included in every group of each study, which meant that you could no longer gauge the outcomes with and without radiotherapy.

One colleague, the leader of the largest Hodgkin's disease clinical trials group in the world, told me privately that he had to include radiotherapy in each group of patients with early disease if he wanted to accrue patients. He needed the cooperation of radiotherapists who often saw these patients first. Ergo, many patients were receiving radiotherapy—needlessly.

This assured that no matter the outcome, radiotherapists would always have a role in the care of patients with Hodgkin's disease— even though our data already indicated that it wasn't necessary and there was reason to believe that exposure to radiation could put patients at risk of future cancers down the road.

The old-guard chemotherapists—the generation who'd tried chemotherapy after World War II—weren't thrilled, either. They didn't like being one-upped and had a hard time letting go of their standard way of doing things—using chemotherapy to palliate, if they used it at all, or using a series of drugs, one at a time—even though this approach didn't work.

Shortly after the MOPP data were published, Professor Rundles from Duke, the one who'd asked me if my patients still spoke to me after I treated them, told a cooperative group meeting that he often got MOPP-like responses with nitrogen mustard alone. You just had to give it over the same long period of time as MOPP, he said. To prove his assertion, he suggested that someone undertake a six-month randomized trial of MOPP versus nitrogen mustard.

I was surprised. Nitrogen mustard had been around a long time, and no one had ever reported those kinds of results. The Southeastern Cancer Study Group ran the study. The version of MOPP it used was cut down to "avoid toxicity," but in the end even the modified dose proved far superior to nitrogen mustard alone.

Not long after these results were available, Dr. Rundles invited me to give grand rounds at Duke to discuss MOPP. When I finished, I looked down from the podium at the now-smiling Wayne Rundles and asked if he remembered wondering if my patients spoke to me posttreatment.

It had become an inside joke between us. He smiled, and I said, "The answer is yes, and for a lot longer."

Despite MOPP's success, there were some problems. One had to do with the meticulous dosing and scheduling of the treatment I had devised. Though I'd spelled it out very carefully, many doctors—in major cancer centers, in academic medical centers, and in private practice—uniformly altered the dosing or the schedule of the drugs.

In 1971, right after I was appointed chief of medicine at the NCI, Barney Clarkson, the chief of the chemotherapy service at Memorial Sloan Kettering, invited me to give a talk on MOPP at its grand rounds. I wasn't likely to get a warm reception, he warned. The hospital hadn't been able to get MOPP to work. It was to be a cross-examination.

I knew MOPP worked, so I accepted. My father, a bank manager in New York City, wanted to know if a nondoctor could attend. He wanted to see his son in action. I was hesitant, knowing I might have to fight a battle with the other doctors, but he sounded so eager that I relented.

The institution's home is an imposing structure that takes up an entire city block from First to York Avenue between Sixty-Seventh and Sixty-Eighth Streets. It had been built on land donated by the Rockefeller family; Laurance Rockefeller essentially owned the place.

We used to hear that the personal wealth of the board members at that time exceeded $5 billion, which was probably a vast underestimate, because Rockefeller alone was worth that much. Its clientele tended toward the rich and the international; its staff was dominated by powerful and well-known cancer surgeons who had popularized the radical mastectomy and set the surgical trends in the country.

Its chemotherapy program had been headed by David Karnofsky, the same man who'd summarily shut me down at the meeting at which I'd presented our MOMP results. Karnofsky was considered by many (especially those at Memorial) the father of chemotherapy and a godlike figure who could do no wrong. He had been involved in the U.S. Army chemical testing program in Aberdeen, Maryland, during World War II, gauging the effects of mustard gas on animals pegged down in the blast field. He and other scientists would run out after the gas exposure and collect the animals for study.

By the time I gave grand rounds at Memorial, he had died of lung cancer, even though he never smoked a day in his life. It was a good bet that his cancer was a result of inhaling all that mustard gas.

His disciples Irwin Krakoff, Joseph Burchenal, and Barney Clarkson considered themselves touched by Karnofsky's greatness. If it didn't originate at Memorial, it couldn't be good, even though most of what they had developed up to that point, in my opinion, hadn't advanced the field much. But Memorial was the largest cancer center in the country and generally considered the best. Going up against them would be a challenge, but by now I was feeling good about my work and relished the chance.

I gave my talk showing the now-astonishing relapse-free survival data and acknowledged the decidedly tepid applause. Then, one after another, several well-known oncologists got up and declared that MOPP didn't work. Clarkson, who was sitting in the front row, let the questions and the accusations roll on for a while. Then he rose to his feet and suggested that something had to be wrong with my data. Joe Burchenal, a leukemia guru, mumbled a comment similar to Karnofsky's earlier criticism. The Memorial physicians' most charitable explanation for MOPP's failure was that we must have only taken on easy-to-treat patients, while Memorial handled the hard cases. I knew the opposite was true.

Then I decided to question them. Directing my gaze at Barney Clarkson, I said, "Barney, tell me exactly how you give the MOPP program here."

I could see the question made him nervous, and for good reason. I suspected that the whole thing had been staged, and at this point, when Barney rose to his feet, I was just supposed to fold. But I wasn't the folding type, and he knew why I was asking the question. Barney described how they administered MOPP at MSKCC. They'd substituted their favorite alkylating agent, thiotepa, at their preferred dose, for nitrogen mustard, without any comparative testing, because they thought it was a better drug and easier to use. Plus, it was "their" drug. Karnofsky, their god, had developed it at Memorial although it was not widely used elsewhere because of erratic effects on the bone marrow. You could never predict what dose would cause marrow toxicity, so they always gave it in low doses. Still, it was the alkylating agent of choice at Memorial.

They'd also cut the dose of procarbazine in half, because it made patients nauseous. And they'd reduced the dose of vincristine drastically because of the risk of nerve damage. They'd also added, at a minimum, an extra two weeks between cycles so that patients would have fully recovered from the toxic effects of the prior dose before they got the next. They gave no thought to the fact that the tumor would have been back on its feet by then, too, apparently. By now, I was more than a little annoyed. I knew exactly why MOPP hadn't worked for them.

"Didn't you read the paper?" I asked. "Don't you realize the importance of the integrity of the four drugs used together at full dose and on schedule?"

I was standing up on the stage behind a podium, looking down at the audience. There was a sort of shocked silence. People generally didn't challenge MSKCC, or Barney Clarkson, for that matter. I could also see that many of the outside physicians in the audience were enjoying the exchange.

They had no rationale for what they were doing. They just didn't believe there was any logic to our original schedules, and they had never developed protocols like ours with a scientific underpinning.

In other words, their version of MOPP was not MOPP at all but a weak imitation they called TOPP (*T* for thiotepa). The problem was, it hadn't been thoroughly devised and tested. More than that, it didn't work. Although patients thought they were getting state-of-the-art treatment, their best shot, they actually weren't.

From my perspective, all our carefully thought-out principles had gone out the window.

After about an hour of this, I blew up.

"Why in God's name have you done this?" I said.

A voice piped up from the audience. "Well, Vince, most of our patients come to us on the subway, and we don't want them to vomit going home."

I was dumbfounded. I addressed the crowd. "If you told those patients that the choice was between being cured and vomiting, or not vomiting and dying, don't you think they might have opted to take a cab?"

That got a good laugh from the audience. I had made my point, I thought.

On my way out of the auditorium, my father caught up with me. He'd shown up late and slipped into the back of the room, unnoticed. We went out to lunch, and I could see he was troubled. He knew being at the NIH meant I must be pretty good, but if what I had done was so great, he asked, why had the doctors at Memorial made such a fuss?

I tried to explain to him that's the way science worked and medicine advanced: we present data for all to see and argue over them. But he knew he'd picked up more than polite professional disagreement in that auditorium. My father, like many, trusted that doctors were an elite group of altruistic people who were somehow a cut above others, both in intelligence and in demeanor. What he'd witness bothered him. He still looked unsettled when I left him.

I didn't discuss with him my feelings about the doctors' having made changes to satisfy their own egos. I didn't think he'd understand it or even believe me. He still thought doctors were above all that. To be honest, I was ashamed at the way the Memorial doctors had behaved. I also felt bad for their patients.

The root of the problem at Memorial was clear to me: The doctors had no confidence that chemotherapy could cure cancer. Or that advanced cancer could be cured at all. Or both. So why make it difficult for patients? If you didn't believe you were denying a patient a curative treatment, then modifications could be made at will. This turned out to be a recurrent theme, well beyond the confines of Memorial.

On top of this, MOPP's potential toxicity scared doctors. The most common response to their fear was to compromise the doses and the schedule. Drugs need to be given with some consideration for the size of the person being treated. Proper dosing is related to blood flow to the kidneys and liver, because these organs are responsible for getting rid of the toxic metabolites of these drugs, and this is best reflected in the total surface area of the body. Put simply, bigger people need bigger doses. A little old lady and a sumo wrestler can't be cured with the same doses. We gave 1.4 mg of vincristine per square meter of body surface area, regardless of what dose that worked out to be.

Most others ended up capping the dose—largely because a group from Stanford University had done it. Led by a well-known chemotherapist, the group at Stanford had repeated MOPP. They'd given it at the proper dose and schedule and with similar results. But they were frightened by vincristine's side effects and recommended that in the future the vincristine dose always be limited to no more than 2 mg. It made no sense to us. Sure, we saw nerve damage from vincristine, but we never saw a patient who didn't recover if he or she went into remission.

We treated a former classmate of mine, a neurosurgeon, who could not work right after MOPP, but a year later he'd fully recovered nerve function and was back in the operating room. Then there was the professional guitarist who couldn't button his own shirt let alone strum the guitar after MOPP. A year later, he was back playing concerts.

The Stanford paper forever fixed the total dose of vincristine at 2 mg, regardless of body size. All future cooperative group studies used the modified vincristine dose and cut other drug doses as well. It was wrong. Most people, if you calculated body surface, needed a larger dose.

If you explained the dose issue to patients, they were willing to risk toxicity. They understood that the payoff was survival. And despite many doctors' concerns about what we were putting them through, the truth is that a person facing imminent death has an entirely different perspective. I had one patient on MOPP confide to me that after each visit to the NIH he left the clinical center by the side door, went to the small decorative pool on the west side of the building, took off his socks and shoes, and waded in the water. I was only dimly aware that the pool existed and completely insensitive to its significance. But he explained it to me: in the book of John in the Bible, there's a reference to pools in Bethesda—a name that in Aramaic means "house of mercy" or "house of grace"—associated with healing. And the NIH was, after all, in Bethesda—albeit not the biblical one. My patient asked me which I thought had worked, MOPP or the pool. I told him we'd take all the help we could get.

Many doctors, on the other hand, seemed less concerned about healing and more worried about being sued or maximizing their income. Patients couldn't push for higher doses if they didn't know that it mattered—and all a doctor had to do was omit that information.

I worked for hours with my friend John Bennett from the University of Rochester Medical Center, a major cancer center in the United States, who said he couldn't make MOPP work, either. I went over the records of all the cases he treated. I even sat in his clinic while he talked to patients. He couldn't get himself to use the word "cure" in front of them, and in all the cases I reviewed, he'd cut the doses and schedules before he ever treated anyone. Like most doctors, he wasn't modifying doses based on a bad experience; he was doing it out of fear of severe side effects.

At a presentation at the Medical Society of the District of Columbia, a local medical oncologist berated me for reporting something that he said didn't work. By now, I knew what to expect and asked how he gave the treatment. He said he couldn't use procarbazine because there was too much nausea associated with it. And he thought vincristine was too toxic, so he just gave nitrogen mustard, "the way you did it," he said, and some steroids. He hadn't, he said, seen anything like what I'd reported. It didn't occur to him that he had reduced MOPP to nothing.

I got a call from a surgeon from the Midwest asking me to take a stage IIIA Hodgkin's patient, a young woman he'd treated with MOPP who'd failed to go into remission. I told him we didn't take previously treated patients, but because he'd described her as a stage IIIA and we'd yet to have a failure in a stage IIIA patient, I asked him how he'd treated her. He said he gave her one cycle of MOPP every three months or so, "as needed." I wondered if he had read our paper at all. I wondered even more why a surgeon was treating a patient with advanced Hodgkin's disease. I felt sorry for that young girl. She'd lost her best chance of being cured.

Things were even worse in Europe, where there were few people even thinking the way we were. An acquaintance from Milan, a pathologist, phoned me after examining the biopsy slides of a young man with advanced Hodgkin's disease who was the son of Eugenio Cefis, an important Italian industrialist.

Cefis wanted me to come over and see his son, who was being cared for by a rheumatologist in Milan. I raised my eyebrows at the mention of the rheumatologist, because such doctors traditionally treat diseases like arthritis, not cancer. I declined. Why put them through the unnecessary expense when I knew he could get good treatment right across town at the Istituto Nazionale dei Tumori, where my friend Gianni Bonadonna had started using MOPP on Hodgkin's disease?

Cefis refused to send his son there. In Italy's class system, the Istituto Nazionale dei Tumori was considered a "guinea pig" institution, a place for ordinary folks who couldn't pay for elite doctors. "Would you be willing to instruct his doctors on the right way to give the MOPP treatment?" Cefis asked me. I agreed but said I needed to see his son's case file. From the information they sent me, it was evident that young Cefis was unusually tall for an Italian, about six feet three. His body surface area meant that he'd need substantial doses of all the drugs in MOPP. When I conferred with his doctor, who spoke good English, so I knew he understood me, I emphasized the importance of the proper dose, based on the patient's size, and the schedule, and even calculated the doses for him.

The reports I received on his case simply listed "MOPP" as his treatment for each of the next six months, without any further details. But by the end of the year, young Cefis was in trouble. Once again, his father asked me to see him. I was scheduled to make an overseas trip for work and had planned to meet my wife in Rome on the way back in three weeks. So I agreed to make a side trip to Milan to see him.

Cefis was a tall, husky, balding man who carried himself with authority and spoke with a quiet voice. His office was elegant—dark wood with deep leather chairs—and very quiet. The blinds were drawn and it was dimly lit, but I could see, just by his demeanor, that Cefis was deeply upset by his son's condition. I told him about what we had been able to do with MOPP at the NCI. He didn't talk much, but he heard me out. He seemed deep in thought.

From his office, I was driven to the private hospital where his son had been admitted. When I walked into the room, I found him surrounded by three doctors. All looked distinguished, gray-haired, and old, dressed in dark suits with white shirts and dark ties. Each one of them carried a cane, though the accessory seemed to be more for appearances' sake than need. It was like a scene from Puccini's *Gianni Schicchi*—each one a wise man pronouncing on the case while the patient lay silent, staring up at the ceiling.

They were visibly horrified at the sight of me. In Italy, the cultural belief, in medicine, was that you had to be old to be a good doctor. I looked even younger than my years and was dressed in a sporty light-blue seersucker suit.

Part of their disdain, I soon realized, was defensive. They had paid no attention to my instructions regarding MOPP. Cefis was a tall young man; his feet hung over the end of his hospital bed. When I reviewed the case notes, I realized that his doctors had ignored my calculations and reduced the doses to token levels—doses so small that they wouldn't have cured a good-sized mouse. He'd essentially been treated just enough to train his tumor cells to become resistant to the drugs.

I was angry with his doctors for their subterfuge, and I led them

out into the hall and told them so. I also told them I was going to
report what they had done to Cefis's father. They were insulted, but I
didn't care. Back in Cefis's office, I explained what had happened.
Again, I suggested he send his son to the Istituto Nazionale dei Tumori, as I had no confidence that his doctors knew what they were
doing. Cefis was noncommittal.

He asked me my fee. I had told him no fee was necessary, but he
insisted, so I suggested $300. He looked surprised and then left the
office for a few minutes. He returned with an envelope. Later, I was
told by the friend who shared dinner with Mary Kay and me that night
that my fee was ridiculously low. He said that Cefis was one of the rich-
est men in Italy. That's why he'd been surprised. He had a slew of
doctors coming through to offer advice, and none had charged less
than $1,000 a visit.

Now I wondered what Cefis really thought of me. Given my appearance and minuscule fee, how could I possibly know what I was
talking about? I left with a feeling of dread for his son. His father's
wealth might, ironically, have cost him his life.

I never heard from Cefis or his son's doctors again. Less than a
year later, my pathologist friend told me that the boy had died.

I had learned, yet again, how a doctor's belief system and the
culture of the medical profession in general could affect the lives of
patients. I was reminded of a comic strip that had recently caused a
stir. In it, a character named Pogo is planted in front of a large mirror
with a shocked look on his face, his hair standing on end and his hat
flying off his head. Around the periphery of this image are the like-
nesses of John Mitchell, Nixon's attorney general, and Bob Haldeman
and John Ehrlichman, Nixon's trusty assistants. The caption reads,
"We have met the enemy, and he is us!"[5]

5

We were making progress at the NCI, but what we were doing still wasn't being used much at other institutions. VAMP and its successors, which fine-tuned the scheduling, among other things, were being used at St. Jude Children's Research Hospital in Memphis, Tennessee. The Roswell Park Cancer Institute in Buffalo, New York, MD Anderson in Houston, Texas, and Memorial Sloan Kettering in Manhattan had adopted the approach as well.

MOPP was a mixed bag. Some doctors used it well; others didn't believe in MOPP and didn't offer it; others modified it, as I've said, without thought for the rationale that we'd used to put it together.

The biggest issue for most doctors—particularly those in private practice, who didn't necessarily have a big staff or the support of a hospital team—was the side effects and the fear of toxicity. They were afraid to use MOPP on their patients, for fear that they wouldn't be able to offer the full care that they needed. However, mortality rates from Hodgkin's disease and leukemia were starting to fall, even with the uneven rollout. And while the public was still unaware that the landscape was shifting in the science of treating cancer (most people still viewed the disease as a complete death sentence), that was about to change, in no small part because of a phone call I received and a patient I didn't want.

In 1969, I was chief of the solid tumor service in the NCI's medicine branch. One day, I got a call from Rita Kelley, a chemotherapist I vaguely knew from the cancer meetings. "Vince, I have a patient who's been diagnosed with inoperable gallbladder cancer," she said. "He's from D.C. He wants to get his treatment near home." She wanted me to take him on as a patient. But my specialty was lymphomas, a pretty far remove from gallbladder cancer. And I knew there was no effective treatment for gallbladder cancer, anyway. "I wish I could help," I said, demurring politely. "But it's not my area." After a brief but cordial chat, we said our goodbyes.

Ten minutes later, my phone rang again. "This is Sidney Farber," said a deep, stentorian voice. *The* Sidney Farber, the Harvard pathologist famous for developing methotrexate, one of the most successful chemotherapy drugs ever discovered.

Farber asked me to take on Rita's patient. Again, I politely declined, explaining once more that I wasn't the right person. Farber paused for a second, then boomed, "You *will* take this patient!" I was a bit surprised, but I wasn't stupid. There was no way I could turn him down.

I couldn't have recognized it then, but this patient, with his unusual and likely untreatable cancer, would have a major impact on the nation's approach to the disease. He had seen some of the most sought-after physicians in the country, including Farber, who wasn't easy to get to. Although I didn't yet know the reason why, obviously this was not just another patient.

A week later, Luke Quinn showed up in my office. He was a wiry man with gray hair, a neatly trimmed mustache, and a fierce scowl. "Hello, Mr. Quinn," I said, reaching out to shake his hand. "It's Colonel Quinn," he snapped. It turned out Quinn had been a U.S. Army

Air Force officer in World War II. It soon became clear that he was used to being in command.

I began to take a routine history, the story the patient tells you about his illness. Then and now, the history and the physical exam are the two most important tools a doctor has at his disposal. They are always available to you, and they don't hurt. If you have experience with the natural history of a disease, how it normally behaves, you can often sense the patient's disease and its stage by using these tools. In this age of rapid scans, I always tell my trainees that if they are unsure of a diagnosis, they need to take the patient's history again and do another physical exam.

"I've been through all of this in Boston," said Quinn testily, cutting me off.

I explained that I needed to do my own history and physical. "When you treat someone with chemotherapy," I explained as patiently as I could, "you need to be aware of the whole person because other problems like high blood pressure or bowel disease can be markedly affected by cancer drugs." I was thinking about Farber's methotrexate, which can tear up the gut in a normal patient and wreak havoc on someone who has an ulcer or colitis. You don't want to be caught off guard.

Quinn glowered at me. Then, reluctantly, he started talking. He'd gone to his regular doctor's office in D.C. when his skin and the whites of his eyes had turned a deep shade of yellow—he had jaundice. But why? Jaundice is a symptom of disease, not a disease itself. Quinn said his doctors had told him that he had obstructive jaundice—a blockage somewhere in his gallbladder that was preventing bile from draining out.

Most of the time, these obstructions are caused by gallstones, which are usually removed surgically.

Quinn's internist had referred him to Claude Welch, at Mass General, for the surgery. Welch was the most famous abdominal surgeon in the country. In those days, some professors at major U.S. medical schools assumed near-godlike status. The Germans called them

Geheimrat professors, a term that signified royalty, and Welch was one of them. When Pope John Paul II was shot in 1981, the Vatican called in Claude Welch to operate. This was another indication that Quinn was a powerfully connected individual, although that still wasn't registering with me.

Quinn's surgery hadn't gone as expected. Instead of gallstones, Welch found a tangled mass of tissue squeezing Quinn's gallbladder. Gallbladder cancer was pretty much a death sentence. Welch excised a piece of it so that a pathologist could confirm the diagnosis, closed Quinn up, and declared him inoperable.

I could surmise the rest. Because Welch couldn't help Quinn, he'd been shuttled over to Rita Kelley to see what she could do for him with chemotherapy. There wasn't much; just one drug, fluorouracil, had a little effect on gallbladder cancer. Kelley knew that Quinn wanted to be treated at home and that his hopes were slim, and she didn't want the case. That's why she'd tried—successfully, as it turned out—to punt him to me.

After Quinn finished his story, I started the physical exam. I listened to his heart and lungs and looked into the back of his eyes with a retinoscope. Next, I examined Quinn's abdomen for a mass I could feel that would indicate the tumor was very advanced. So far, everything was routine.

Then I slipped my hands under Quinn's arms, to examine his armpits, home of the axillary lymph nodes, a cluster of glands that can provide clues to what's going on in the body. Normally, these glands are so small that you can't feel them. If the patient has an infection, they might become engorged with white blood cells and tender to the touch. If they're full of tumor cells escaped from solid tumors, such as those of breast or lung cancer, the nodes tend to feel hard. When they're full of tumor cells from lymphomas, they feel rubbery.

When I felt Quinn's axillary lymph nodes, something wasn't right. The lymph nodes in both axillae were enlarged and rubbery. Gallbladder cancer can do a lot of bad things to you, but most of them happen in the liver; the cancer usually stays pretty local. I'd never seen or heard of a case with swollen glands as far away as the axillary nodes, especially in both axillae, because they are anatomically disconnected. He appeared to have a generalized lymphadenopathy, a disease affecting lymph nodes everywhere. Apparently, none of his doctors had noticed this before. It could be I just hadn't seen enough of gallbladder cancer. But Quinn's lymph nodes made me wonder what was going on. Lymphomas, which I had seen plenty of, can cause enlarged lymph nodes throughout the body, including in the axillary nodes and even around the gallbladder. Was it possible that what Welch saw was not gallbladder cancer but lymphoma wrapped around the gallbladder? That could have caused the obstruction that had led to jaundice.

I told Quinn that I had some questions about his diagnosis. He was annoyed. "I just want to get on with my treatment," he snapped. I wondered if anyone had told him about the grim prognosis for gallbladder cancer. Quinn had arrived with his biopsy slides in hand, a matter of course when a doctor is sending a patient to someone else. Now I asked him for them. Still angry, he handed me the slides, and I sent him out to the waiting room while I walked the slides over to the office of Costan Berard, my favorite pathologist at the NCI. Cos was a trim, stern-looking guy with short, graying hair. He talked in a clipped manner and loved to lecture you about what he was looking at. Everything about Cos was precise, and I loved his off-the-cuff tutorials. I learned a lot about lymphoma pathology from him.

A good cancer doctor never wants to be too far from his pathologist. They are the ones who make the diagnosis, and it is not easy. Errors are not uncommon. We already knew, for example, that about 6 percent of patients were erroneously diagnosed with a lymphoma. But I trusted Cos and thought he was the best pathologist I had ever worked with.

I told Berard I had reservations about the diagnosis and handed him the box. One by one, he took out the slides, held them up toward the ceiling light, and studied them. Then, silently, he slipped each slide under his microscope. As he was eyeing the last slide, he paused, one eye still glued to the barrel. "I think there might be a compression artifact," he said.

A compression artifact indicates that in removing tissue from a patient, the surgeon has inadvertently squeezed it, which morphs the shape of the cells, possibly making it hard to differentiate one kind of cancer cell from another. Gallbladder cancer cells are compact and elliptical. Lymphoma cells, like the lymphocyte cells they arise from, are round. Compressing them, however, can make them assume an elliptical shape—like that of cancerous gallbladder cells, in fact.

It wasn't just the compression artifact that had given Berard pause. Lymphoma cells can distort the shape of the lymph node from which they arose, partially erasing its architecture. But a good pathologist can usually still recognize the outline of a node, even with the naked eye, by simply holding the slide up to the light. When Berard had done this with Quinn's slides, he was pretty sure he'd seen traces of lymph nodes.

It was possible that the Boston pathologist was aware of Welch's impression that Quinn had gallbladder cancer and had been swayed by it when he read the slides. Cos, unimpeded by bias, saw something quite different.

I wasn't entirely surprised, either. I had a strong hunch that Quinn had a lymphoma, not cancer of the gallbladder. But we needed another biopsy to be sure. I wasn't looking forward to suggesting it to Quinn, whom I'd left fuming in the waiting room. I returned to my office and called Quinn in to give him the news. I could see the wheels turning in his head as he glared at me, trying to decide whether to get up and leave. I'd come highly recommended by Rita Kelley, but I was young, just thirty-four, and looked it. I was a bit surprised when Quinn agreed.

It was a good thing that he did. The new biopsy showed, without a doubt, that Quinn had non-Hodgkin's lymphoma, or NHL, the awkward non-name we give to all lymphomas that are not Hodgkin's disease. Quite by accident, and no thanks to me, Quinn had landed in exactly the right place.

We were working on a new drug combination for non-Hodgkin's lymphoma, C-MOPP, in which we substituted cyclophosphamide for nitrogen mustard, its cousin. The early results were impressive. About 40 percent of patients with the aggressive form of this lymphoma were staying in remission beyond two years, which until now had been unheard of. We were focused on our Hodgkin's work and had not yet published the C-MOPP results, so they were not widely known. But it looked as if we were on our way to curing another intractable cancer with chemotherapy. Treating Quinn for gallbladder cancer would have done little or nothing, and he would have died. But now he had a shot.

We admitted Quinn to the hospital and treated him for three months. It was a long three months. The nurses hated him. They thought he was the most arrogant, demanding patient they'd ever seen. He wanted the second bed in his room kept empty so he could conduct important business, even though we needed the beds and had no private rooms. On a ward full of sick patients, he demanded service immediately, leaning on his call button until a nurse appeared. And he complained bitterly about the food. One of the things that enraged him the most was when people—including me—forgot to address him as Colonel Quinn. No one could ever recall him saying thank you. Quinn should have been more polite, because those nurses and the doctors they worked with were giving him an incredible gift. By the time he was discharged, all signs of his tumor had disappeared. He'd gone from a certain death sentence to having a fighting chance.

So why was this gruff, unpleasant patient so important in launching the war on cancer? It wasn't him; it was the people he knew.

It's a sign of how politically naive I was that it never occurred to me to wonder how Quinn had ended up as a patient of the famous Claude Welch, for something that appeared to be garden-variety gallstones, and then Sidney Farber. That's like showing up for a pickup game with Larry Bird and Michael Jordan as your teammates. If I had thought about it, I would have concluded that Quinn had to be very well connected. But I didn't think about it. Not until I discovered that Quinn was a friend and employee of the socialite and philanthropist Mary Lasker.

The first time I met Mary was in 1969 at the National Advisory Cancer Council (NACC) meetings. Each NIH institute had an advisory council; the NCI had the NACC. Mary was quite different from the other council members, most of whom were physicians and men who wore dark suits and ties with white shirts. With brown hair coiffed in a perfect bouffant, a mink coat slung carelessly over her chair, and perfectly applied makeup, Mary had the appearance of a lightweight socialite with too much time on her hands. Except that even when she was eyeing herself in her compact mirror, which she did frequently, she was clearly listening.

I had a vague sense that she'd been involved in the politics of medical research, but I didn't know to what extent. I sensed that many people at the NCI were afraid of her. I consequently learned that she was very much a heavyweight, despite her appearance, and, indeed, more than a little scary.

Mary was the widow of Albert Lasker, an advertising magnate who'd made a fortune off the revenue from Lucky Strike cigarettes. Albert Lasker was her second husband. Her first was Paul Reinhardt, owner of Reinhardt Galleries in New York City, whom she married in 1926, three years out of Radcliffe College, and divorced in 1934 because of his alcoholism.

She first met Albert Lasker at social gatherings in the spring of 1939. She was living on $25,000 a year. During conversations with Mary, he became impressed with her attention to detail, how she made and spent her money, and her many interests. By that time, she'd already been involved in drives for national health insurance, birth control, psychoanalysis, and preventive medicine.

He thought it amazing that she got so much out of so little. In June 1940, they were married. Albert said he'd married her for her money. For a time, Mary insisted on keeping separate bank accounts because she wanted to pay her own way. But she was interested in so many causes and didn't have enough money to support herself and her passions. She found herself saying, "No, sorry, I don't have the money for this," to those who came to solicit her help in the palatial home she shared with Albert.

Albert was a very rich Chicago businessman. He lived on a 350-acre estate just outside Chicago and kept a 150-foot yacht on Lake Michigan that required twenty-four crewmen to operate. He wasn't interested in health issues the way Mary was. According to Mary, he was afraid of illness and doctors and didn't want to know details about disease. But he was embarrassed by her "poverty," and he persuaded her to accept his million-dollar gift so that she could support her causes, which, at that time, included health insurance and cancer and tuberculosis research.

He also told her that to get those kinds of things done, she didn't need his kind of money. "You need federal money, and I'll show you how to get it." One of the first things she learned was there was no point in going to agency heads to ask them to ask for more money or to establish new programs. You needed to aim higher. You went to the president himself, or you went to the congressional committees that supplied the money.

She wasted no time. In the fall of 1941, through the good offices of her friend Anna Rosenberg, who was close to Eleanor Roosevelt, she wangled an invitation for an overnight stay at the White House and had dinner with President Roosevelt and lunch the next day with leaders of the Public Health Service. Though her interests changed over time, her determination never did.

Mary soon racked up an impressive list of accomplishments. In 1942, the Laskers created the Albert and Mary Lasker Foundation, which annually recognizes some of the top U.S. medical researchers and clinicians with the Lasker Award—frequently referred to as the American Nobel Prize. Indeed, many winners go on to receive the Nobel for research first recognized by the Laskers.

In 1945, when the American Cancer Society was known as the American Society for the Control of Cancer, Lasker and her husband agreed to underwrite a campaign to raise money for the society if it would change its name to the American Cancer Society and put at least 25 percent of the money raised into cancer research. At this point, the society didn't have much money, and none of it went toward research. What resources it had went to helping cancer patients cope with their diagnoses—helping them find the right doctors and hospice-like resources, for instance. The Laskers also insisted that the organization change its policy and appoint laypeople to fill half of its board seats, which at that point had been doled out only to doctors.

Mary also played a role in what would turn out to be a Nobel Prize–winning discovery. In 1946, the microbiologist Selman Waksman published a paper on streptomycin, a new class of antibiotic that appeared to be effective against certain microbes that were not vulnerable to penicillin. Mary, who was not a scientist, pointed out to Waksman that the drug had had some effect against tuberculosis. There were no useful drugs for the disease at the time, and Waksman himself, along with most of organized medicine, initially thought the results not promising enough to pursue. Mary's instincts said otherwise. She persuaded Waksman and the Merck pharmaceutical company to support tests of streptomycin against TB. By 1952, the widespread use of streptomycin resulted in cutting mortality from TB in half—only a few years after the drug's discovery. You might say she helped him win the Nobel Prize, which he received that same year for developing the tuberculosis cure.

Meanwhile, Mary and her good friend Florence Mahoney, wife of the publisher of *The Miami News*, put a full-court press on the White House and Congress to expand the National Institutes of Health by establishing new institutes within it. Mary had Congress figured out. Her mantra was that Congress wouldn't be generous in funding a concept—something like "biological research." But propose funding for an institute named after a feared disease, and you'd make progress. Their incessant lobbying, with Albert's assistance and financial support, helped to create the National Cancer Institute, the National Heart Institute, the National Eye Institute, the National Institute of Mental Health, the National Institute of Dental and Craniofacial Research, the National Institute of Arthritis and Metabolic Diseases, the National Institute on Aging, and the National Institute of Child Health and Human Development.

Organized medicine and academia believed that independent investigators should be funded to pursue their own research interests, wherever they led. Mary's funding, however, came with strings attached. When she supported projects, she did so only when there was a specific goal, such as curing tuberculosis—or cancer. Mary knew the value of independent research but believed that in order to transfer exciting laboratory discoveries to the clinic, you also needed well-funded, organized programs. The NIH, which brought brainpower and labs and patients under one roof, was the place to do this in her opinion. But it had no interest in anything but supporting basic research.

The American Cancer Society was different. Lane Adams, the executive vice president of the ACS from 1960 until 1986, was a close friend of Mary's. The Laskers had pressed the ACS to support focused research, which it was now doing. And it supported her demands for more money from the federal government.

Mary's influence continued throughout the 1950s and the 1960s, and she was at the height of her power during the time we were developing the first cancer cures at the National Cancer Institute. That's when Luke Quinn became her influential lieutenant.

Mary was not above a little sleuthing to be sure she was pushing the right levers in Congress. She needed a pair of eyes and ears on Capitol Hill that could not be traced directly to her. Luke Quinn, who had been the air force military liaison to Congress during World War II, was that man. Members of Congress thought he represented the American Cancer Society, but in reality he was a lobbyist who, by agreement with the ACS, reported directly to Mary. Mary Lasker paid his salary behind the scenes.

His job was to gather intelligence on members of Congress. Those who favored her initiatives were introduced to Mary's wealthy friends, who made contributions to their campaigns. Those who were neutral were subjected to Mary's full-court press, which usually included visits with distinguished researchers and Washington power brokers. Those who were hostile were subjected to what Mary referred to as "the Sword," an organization called Citizens' Committee for the Conquest of Cancer. Headed by Solomon Garb, a pharmacology professor at the University of Colorado, the group was essentially a letter-writing organization, with branches in every state, that harassed members of Congress who wouldn't support Mary's proposals. As a result, many of Mary's opponents rethought their positions.

When Quinn got sick, Mary had used her connections to get to Welch, under the protective wing of Sidney Farber. And when Quinn's apparently hopeless case suddenly looked less hopeless, it got her attention. That was important because Mary Lasker had money, influence on Capitol Hill, and a reputation as perhaps the most powerful advocate for biomedical research that Washington had ever seen.

Ongoing public concern about cancer made it an ideal disease for Mary to attack. Mary's personal experience underscored her interest, too: Albert Lasker died of pancreatic cancer in 1952, leaving her his fortune. Mary immediately stepped up her efforts on cancer.

Mary had been impressed by the antimalaria-drug-screening program in World War II as well as the information on nitrogen mustard that emanated from the Chemical Warfare Service, for instance. Through a massive screening program, effective drugs had been found to treat malaria. This had an enormously positive effect on the war effort in the Pacific region, where malaria was rampant.

The Chemical Warfare Service, headed by Cornelius "Dusty" Rhoads, a doctor on leave from Memorial Hospital for Cancer and Allied Diseases in New York (now Memorial Sloan Kettering Cancer Center), was in the Office of Medical Research. That's where the information on nitrogen mustard, a derivative of the war gas phosgene and one of the drugs in MOPP, had come from.

What she saw was that given a project and some money, scientists could work in a focused way to solve a problem. Why, she wondered, weren't we doing more of that work toward finding new drugs that worked against cancer?

In 1952, Mary urged Congress to find more drugs for cancer. She pressed it to provide funds to the National Cancer Institute to set up a national screening program for cancer drugs. Congress had initially given the NCI $1 million toward the effort.

In 1954, at Mary's urging, Congress held hearings to determine the progress the cancer institute had made with the screening program. The answer: not much. Frustrated by the NCI's foot-dragging, in 1955, Mary pressed Congress to provide another $5 million to the NCI, this time with a mandate to develop an actual drug-screening program. The cancer institute had no choice but to set up the program.

The National Cancer Institute was not happy about this challenge to its own initiatives, but after much cajoling by Mary and Congress, and an additional infusion of funds, the NCI did what was asked of it. It was this program that Dave Rall had been referring to when he tried to sell me on the NCI, years earlier, when I was still a medical student.

The program was hugely controversial at the NCI. Few thought that drugs had any chance of curing a complex problem like cancer. Many thought that money invested in random screening was a waste. To make matters worse, the institute decided to use contracts and not the established way of doling out money—Research Project or R01 grants—to fund the program. This put it squarely on Mary Lasker's side of the debate about applied versus basic research. Contracts are used when you want to hire somebody to come up with a solution to a problem. Grants allow researchers to roam more widely, to see what they can learn—not to solve an immediate problem. Grant-funded research often helps solve problems years or decades later, but it is not intended to meet practical goals. It's all about the pursuit of knowledge.

While research contracts had been effective for the Defense Department, the NCI's use of them was a first at the NIH, and it was not met with enthusiasm. Research supported by contracts was—and

still is—considered second-rate. But despite the resistance from organized medicine, the NCI, the NIH, academia, and the American
Medical Association (AMA), Mary prevailed. And out of this program came the drugs used to create VAMP and MOMP and MOPP
and C-MOPP and all the other drugs we'd been working on in the
lab and in the clinic.

By 1964, Mary was at it again. Impressed by several papers that
reported virus particles in some patients with cancer, Mary persuaded
Congress to provide the NCI with another $5 million to set up the
Special Virus Cancer Program (SVCP) to look for viral causes of
cancer. Supported by research contracts, it was almost as controversial as the cancer-drug-screening program.

Now I understood why Mary was on the National Advisory
Cancer Council and why people were afraid of her. Somehow, this
demure, beehived socialite could circumvent all the conventions of
medicine and medical research, no matter how loud the protests, and
she could get Congress to do things her way.

Mary was excited by Quinn's startling recovery, and she was savvy
enough to understand its significance. We could now get at those
errant tumor cells that escaped into the bloodstream, beyond the reach
of surgery or radiation. Our work had proven that the right combination of cancer drugs could cure some types of patients with advanced
cancer. She thought that with a massive research effort to strengthen
the approaches being used to combat leukemia, Hodgkin's disease,
and non-Hodgkin's lymphoma, we could cure cancer.

Mary was guided by two principles in setting priorities for select-
ing areas for support. First, the medical problem had to be of major
concern to the American people, and, second, there must be some
evidence that a change had occurred in the field that could be exploited by an infusion of resources.

Polls had shown that the disease the American public feared most
was cancer. And Mary saw, in Quinn's recovery, and the work we had
done, reason to believe that the necessary research change had occurred to justify taking the disease head-on. Mary decided that the

country that had put a man on the moon eight years after President Kennedy made it a national mission was ready to declare war on cancer.

In April 1970, Mary persuaded her good friend the Texas Democratic senator Ralph Yarborough, who was chair of the Committee on Labor and Public Welfare, to pass a Senate resolution to create the National Panel of Consultants on the Conquest of Cancer.

Because the president—Richard Nixon—was a Republican and Mary a tried-and-true Democrat, she needed bipartisan support. She prevailed on Yarborough to appoint her friend the wealthy Republican businessman Benno C. Schmidt to be the chairman of the panel on the conquest of cancer. He already had a connection with cancer research: he was chairman of Memorial Sloan Kettering's powerful board of managers. She backed him up by arranging for Sidney Farber to be named co-chairman. The twenty-four-member panel of consultants also included Luke Quinn—and, of course, Mary. Most of the rest of the panel were well-known doctors and scientists who were advocates for more support for cancer research.

The panel issued "The Yarborough Report" in just six months and made far-reaching recommendations, including that an independent agency—a national cancer authority—be established "whose mission is defined by statute to be the conquest of cancer."

The National Cancer Institute would be transferred to this new agency. This authority would be headed by an administrator appointed by the president with advice and consent of the Senate, and he should report directly to the president and present his budgets and programs to the Office of Management and Budget (OMB) directly, bypassing the NIH entirely.

The report also called for a national comprehensive cancer plan for vanquishing the disease as promptly as possible. It recommended a substantial increase in funding for cancer research from $180 million in 1971 to $400 million in 1972, reaching $800 million to $1 billion by 1976. It also stipulated that the financing of the program not result in cuts to other health programs. Finally, it recommended that the approval for anticancer drugs be moved from the FDA to the new cancer authority.

Luke Quinn, whom I still saw for checkups, told me he and Mary had actually written most of the report for Yarborough's staff. Yarborough introduced the legislation, but he was defeated in his reelection bid in 1970. Senator Edward Kennedy succeeded to the chairmanship and introduced the panel's recommendations as new legislation for the Ninety-Second Congress.

Quinn was a busy man in those days. In addition to writing the bill itself, he orchestrated the hearings, set the agenda, and selected the people who would testify. Remarkable, really, because he was not a Senate staff member.

He pumped me with questions about cancer statistics, breakthroughs, and other areas to cover in hearings, and he often asked me who I thought should testify in favor of the bill. He met with each one for a dress rehearsal to judge his or her fitness to testify. Most of the people whose names I submitted, including Tom Frei, were ignored in favor of those in Mary's entourage. Quinn explained to me that there was an art to testifying before Congress and most academics were unsuited because they were reluctant to put emotion into their testimony, to exaggerate and inflate as a means to an end. He needed flamboyant witnesses.

He never asked me to be a witness, either, suspecting I was sympathetic to the NIH position that moving the NCI out of the NIH was a bad idea—or maybe thinking I was not sufficiently flamboyant.

I was not sure if that was a compliment or not.

The Nixon administration did not immediately embrace the Kennedy bill. Nixon proposed much more conservative alternative legislation that called for increasing funding to just under $100 million for cancer research and no organizational changes. And he wasn't thrilled about Ted Kennedy's involvement. Nixon sent word through his channels that he might support the proposed new cancer act if Kennedy was not a sponsor. Kennedy and Mary Lasker were close friends. She took it upon herself to approach him with this news and asked him to withdraw as sponsor. He agreed, and Senator Pete Domenici of New Mexico introduced the bill.

It drew immediate attacks from academia, the NIH, and the AMA, all of whom opposed it. Kennedy held hearings on the bill, and many others in the administration and scientific organizations took that opportunity to express their opposition. They argued that money could not buy ideas and that funding cancer research to this degree would siphon money away from other institutes and research. They also argued that if you gave the cancer institute such largesse, every other institute would want the same treatment, which was clearly not feasible. All predicted the downfall of the NIH, medical schools, and research as we knew them if we went through with a national initiative to cure cancer.

In an eloquent letter to Senator Kennedy in March 1971 after the hearings had ended, Benno Schmidt made the case for Domenici's bill—now known as the National Cancer Act—and effectively responded to all the arguments. Schmidt's letter quoted testimony from Carl Baker, then the acting director of the NCI, before the National Panel of Consultants on the Conquest of Cancer. Benno quoted it, he said, "because it gave a better picture of the nature of the problems" than did the testimony of others in the administration. Baker compared the proposed cancer program to air defense in the Battle of Britain, the Manhattan Project, and the moon shot.

Baker—via Schmidt—won the debate. His testimony made it clear that the existing small grant program, with all its bureaucracy, was not the way to go. Meanwhile, Mary's allies swung into action with letter-writing campaigns, bombarding senators who opposed the bill—and with what turned out to be the coup de grâce.

Mary had many ways to put public pressure on Congress when she needed to. One was to tap her good friend the wildly popular advice columnist Ann Landers, whose column was syndicated in newspapers nationwide and had an estimated ninety million readers, for help.

On April 20, 1971, Ann Landers wrote a letter to her readers. It was titled "Advice for the Millions." She began, "Dear readers, if you're looking for a laugh today, you'd better skip Ann Landers. If you want to be part of an effort that might save millions of lives—maybe your own—please stay with me." She went on to cite statistics about cancer and pointed out that in 1969 for every man, woman, and child in the United States the U.S. government spent $125.00 on the war in Vietnam, $19.00 on the space program, $19.00 in foreign aid, and $0.89 on cancer research.

She pointed out to her readers that a bill would soon come before the Senate that would call for the establishment of the National Cancer Authority. She went on to say, "Today you have the opportunity to be a part of the mightiest offensive against a single disease in the history of our country. If enough citizens let their Senators know they want Bill S34 passed, it will pass. I urge each and every person who reads this column to write to his two Senators at once—or better yet, send telegrams . . . Your message need consist of only three words: 'Vote for S34.' And sign your name please." She closed with "Thanks— and God bless."

In the next few days, the Senate was deluged with more letters and telegrams than it had ever received. Senate secretaries wore signs that said "Impeach Ann Landers," they were so overloaded. But secretly, they loved the idea. The bill passed with only one vote against it, cast by Senator Gaylord Nelson of Wisconsin.

But the battle was not over. The bill originated in the Senate but had to pass in the House. The House health subcommittee was chaired by Congressman Paul Rogers of Florida. He was well connected to the NIH and academia. Luke Quinn had little influence over Rogers, who, like the NIH, was concerned about the proposal to remove the NCI from the NIH and transfer drug approval authority from the FDA to the NCI.

The committee held hearings on the various proposals. Hostile witnesses said removing cancer research from the NIH would result in a loss of coordination among the various related institutes, crippling research. They cautioned that the NIH would face similar "threats of separation," as they put it, with other disease areas.

These objections, of course, were straw men. There was never any coordination of research efforts among the institutes at that time, and very little research relevant to cancer was carried on outside the NCI. But the arguments, largely coming from academic institutions and the NIH, were effective. After the hearings, Paul Rogers and the panel chair, Benno Schmidt, met and reached a compromise.

A new bill was offered that kept the NCI in the NIH but gave the NCI a separate budget. The bill established the President's Cancer Panel to oversee the cancer effort, and it said the panel's chair would report directly to the president—not to the NIH director.

The NCI director would also be a presidential appointee. To assuage the NIH, the bill made the NIH director a presidential appointment as well. And it recommended a significant increase in funding.

On December 23, 1971, the cancer act was signed as a "Christmas gift to the nation" by President Richard Nixon, two years after Quinn had walked into my office with the wrong diagnosis.[1] It was a victory for Lasker and a victory for the nation, which was still terrified—justifiably—of this disease. The biggest disappointment for Mary had been the failure to transfer authority for approval of cancer drugs from the FDA to the NCI, a failure that would dog the National Cancer Program well into the future. I'll tell you just how in a later chapter.

But we had made a start. And with the passage of Mary's bill, cancer research was on the fast track. We had money. We had an institute with a reasonable amount of independence. And we had a goal. The national war on cancer had begun.

6

> Boots on the Ground: Having boots on the ground in an
> area means to have soldiers there in order to control what is
> happening . . . especially to prevent opposing forces from
> carrying out and launching operations from there.
> —*Urban Dictionary*, definition no. 2

For a long time, I was irritated by the phrase "the war on cancer." It came about because the National Cancer Act was passed when Vietnam was still ongoing and war and body counts were analogies that came easily to journalists looking for an economical turn of phrase.

That said, there are some apt war analogies for the way that the effort against cancer unfurled, and "boots on the ground" is one of them. The phrase refers to the process of delivering soldiers to the area of conflict and organizing them in a system rational for both assault and defense.

It takes expertise and a great deal of reasoning to make a system efficient. We rely on experienced generals for the strategic planning of such things. It's critical, obviously, that the plan be right. Lives depend on it.

I chose definition number two, above, because it encompasses an added aspect of boots on the ground: defense of one's position. The soldiers in question here have a dual role: their own combat mission, but also the job of preventing opposing forces from taking over and assuming the position they've acquired.

When the war on cancer began, the job at hand was to get boots on the ground in an organized fashion, one that optimized the assault plan and protected our turf. But it was messier, far messier, than anyone had thought it would be. And there was a constant pushback from those who'd opposed the war on cancer and were not interested in seeing it succeed, which necessitated strong defensive posture.

Despite chemotherapy's rough start, and despite considerable pessimism in the field, we'd provided "proof of principle"—proof that chemotherapy could cure advanced cancer. It was not pointless cruelty, as the naysayers had insisted. People who would otherwise be dead were leaving the hospital and resuming their lives. This had happened because of a commitment to basic research in the field of drug development.

In late September 1972, we learned that we were not the only ones who believed in chemotherapy. I got word that I would share the Lasker Award with Frei, Freireich, and a handful of other pioneers in the development of curative chemotherapy for cancer. The citation read that I was being honored for an "outstanding contribution to the concept of combination therapy in the treatment of Hodgkin's disease." It was a heady validation.

I was thirty-seven and chief of the medicine branch at the NCI. I'd come a long way from the med student who thought he'd carry a black bag and make house calls after graduation. Instead, I now spent most of my waking hours on 12 West at the NIH Clinical Center, treating cancer. I owned a black bag; every new graduate of my era did. But it sat in my closet, untouched.

In 1965, when I'd completed my stint as a clinical associate, half of all children with childhood leukemia had been entering complete remission and returning to normal lives. Now we knew that half of those remissions turned out to be cures. By 1970, the cure rate had crept up to 50 percent—this in a disease that had once been 100 percent fatal and that had claimed its tiniest victims in gruesome fashion. In 1965, 80 percent of all patients with advanced Hodgkin's disease were going into complete remissions and returning to normal. Two-thirds of these cases had turned out to be cures. By 1970, 70 percent of all patients with all stages of Hodgkin's disease were curable.

The news wasn't as good for other cancers. We had a long way to go, but there was no question that we had found what cancer treatment had long been missing—a therapy capable of chasing cells that had escaped the primary tumor into the bloodstream, lymph channels, and other organs. We just had to find the right drugs and how to combine them with the existing therapies in order to vanquish the other cancers.

It was a big "just," but not an insurmountable one, it seemed, especially now that the nation had declared "war" on the disease.

On 12 West, with the money provided by the new National Cancer Act, we were building on what we'd started—expanding the reach of combination chemotherapy as a treatment. The medicine branch was an incredibly powerful research tool. We had twenty-six beds. We didn't have to apply for grant support for our work; it was written into our budgets. Patients needed no insurance and were admitted free of charge. We could draw the patients we needed for studies from all over the country, because we could pay for their travel and put them and their families up at government expense at the Town and Country Inn.

This was the ideal way to do clinical research. All the roadblocks that make it difficult to translate an experiment with mice in a lab to a clinical experiment with humans—the inability to travel, lack of money, and insufficient insurance—were gone. We were unfettered, limited only by what was between our ears.

I had begun to assemble my senior staff. The nicknamer extraordinaire George Canellos, my former fellow clinical associate who had once mocked the MOMP program Moxley and I had put together, had returned from England. And he had become a believer. Two of my trainees, Bob Young and Bruce Chabner, after a year of training at Yale, had returned as well. Soon, one of our former research associates, Phil Schein, joined us after a year of training in Boston. With each class of clinical associates that passed through the clinical center, the clutch of doctors who believed in the potential for curing cancer grew.

The success with Hodgkin's disease had given us momentum. The larger message from the early studies was that drugs could cure advanced cancers such as leukemia, Hodgkin's disease, and diffuse large B-cell lymphoma (DLBCL). The next step was to use chemotherapy to treat the more common solid tumors, but we needed to develop a master plan. The room with four blackboards in which the Society of Jabbering Idiots had flourished wasn't available anymore. But we re-created it the best we could.

Over the course of the next two years, we spent hours hammering out study protocols in the big solarium on the twelfth floor. One wall of the solarium comprised windows that faced out over the NIH campus. Clinical associates, patients, and their families tended to gather in the solarium to enjoy the lounge chairs and the view, and they regularly drifted through the meetings. Sometimes, they stopped to listen for a while.

As chief of the branch, I led the discussions, but all participants spoke when they wanted to and were welcome to grab a piece of chalk to scribble on the portable blackboard on wheels we used. We were united in our belief we could cure cancer with drugs, but we had very different personalities, and discussions could get loud and somewhat cantankerous. Our clinical associates often thought we were fighting. We weren't, not really. Our loudness was a measure of our enthusiasm. George nicknamed everyone with biting accuracy. Bob Young became "Dr. Exclamation Point," because he spoke mostly in forceful declarative sentences. Phil Schein became "Dr. Greed," because he wanted to be part of every study. Bruce Chabner became "Sleepy" (of *Snow White and the Seven Dwarfs* fame) because he had the habit of nodding off until a key word was mentioned, at which point he'd startle awake and pitch in with some clever idea. George had many nicknames for me—only some of which he used in my presence. His favorite was "Rockville's Rossano Brazzi," because, he said, I looked like the Italian actor. I didn't believe him but didn't want to ask the *real* meaning.

I had already set up two Hodgkin's trials. One tested the need for maintenance therapy on MOPP. If patients who received no further treatment did as well as those who got maintenance treatment, it would validate our contention that patients who entered complete remission were cured. Bob Young took that study over. We also outlined a controversial study that would compare MOPP alone with radiation therapy alone in early-stage disease. I knew we'd take heat for that one; not only was radiotherapy considered effective for early-stage disease, but radiotherapists continued to argue that it was heretical, even unethical, to totally omit X-ray treatment for early-stage disease.

But we wanted to expand. The real question of the day was whether what we learned with Hodgkin's disease and childhood leukemia could be applied to the more common cancers, referred to as solid tumors. Of particular interest was the application of Skipper's inverse rule. That is, if a program worked to some degree in an advanced stage of a common cancer, where many cancer cells were present, would it cure patients who presented with early disease, no visible cancer after surgery, but a high risk of recurrence because cancer cells had, in most cases, slipped the leash?

There were several common cancers, like breast and colon cancer, that often presented with what appeared to be early disease. In breast cancer, for instance, 90 percent of patients presented with localized disease. Many went home after surgery, being told the surgeon had "gotten it all." But few were cured. Adjuvant chemotherapy—the use of chemotherapy as an adjunct to surgery or radiotherapy—would involve treating patients who were apparently free of disease after surgery. It was, heretofore, a no-no. The first step we'd need to take, we decided, was to develop good programs in patients with these cancers who already had advanced visible disease.

One of the first we decided to take on was advanced ovarian

cancer. Bob Young led the study and published the results, which introduced the first combination chemotherapy program to treat that disease. We also had a new drug in the pipeline that destroyed the islet cells of the pancreas, the cells that produce insulin. It was a cousin of BCNU, the exploding drug I'd worked with as a clinical associate. These drugs were called nitrosoureas. Our chemists were isolating a whole bunch of them to see if they could make a better drug. This one called streptozotocin had the surprising effect of attacking the islet cells. In mice, it caused diabetes. Most thought that this was a bad side effect, obviously. But we reasoned it might prove useful for insulinoma, a type of pancreatic cancer that derived from those cells. (And this drug didn't explode.) In its malignant form, insulinoma not only grew and metastasized but secreted copious amounts of insulin, putting patients at risk for diabetic coma. The only other drug that worked against it was 5-fluorouracil, and it was only marginally effective. Phil Schein directed that study (it worked). Not only did it stop insulin production in these patients, but it also controlled the growth of the tumor. All future protocols that involved endocrine cancer were run by Phil.

In a short time, we had exciting studies in Hodgkin's disease, non-Hodgkin's lymphoma, ovarian cancer, and the endocrine cancer known as malignant insulinoma. And we were running a number of early drug trials, not only doing the phase I and II studies but also studying the pharmacology of these drugs—their chemistry, their structure, what they attacked, and how the body metabolized them. Bruce Chabner, our most skilled clinical pharmacologist, managed these studies.

George Canellos and I set up the CMF protocol (CMF for the drug combination—cyclophosphamide, methotrexate, and fluorouracil) along the lines of MOPP. We used this to treat patients with advanced breast cancer and produced the best results in breast cancer that had so far been seen.[1]

But we had a problem. We could assemble enough patients with advanced disease to test CMF, but to do an adjuvant study—that is, of chemotherapy in conjunction with surgery—we needed breast cancer

patients post-surgery. Because we had no surgical breast cancer program at the NCI, we didn't have access to these patients. We were
going to need the cooperation of surgeons. But, like radiotherapists,
they were loath to let the newbies on the block, medical oncologists,
enter what had long been their territory.

First we tried to persuade the major cancer centers in the United
States—MD Anderson and Memorial Sloan Kettering—to run the
study. Neither place would touch it. Their surgeons thought we
were crazy. Who gave drugs to patients who appeared to be free of
disease when some would never develop a recurrence if left alone?
(Never mind that for a large number of patients, their cancer would
recur, and they would die as a result.)

We had to go overseas to find surgeons who'd take the leap. Paul
Carbone had many European contacts and eventually persuaded
Umberto Veronesi, the flamboyant director of the Istituto Nazionale
dei Tumori in Milan (and a well-known breast cancer surgeon), to consider it. Veronesi was a European dynamo. Patients with breast cancer
came from all over Italy to see him. The Istituto Nazionale dei Tumori
was operating on more than a thousand patients a year with localized
breast cancer (meaning breast cancer that had not visibly spread beyond the site of the primary tumor).

Veronesi was impeccably polite, fluent in three languages, handsome, rich, and drove fast cars. On a visit to the institute, I asked him
how long it would take me to drive my rental car to the Lake Como
area from Milan. He paused and looked at me for a moment,
thoughtfully. "For you, an hour, for me, thirty minutes," he said in all
seriousness. Getting him on board would be a major coup.

Veronesi sent Gianni Bonadonna, his medical oncologist, to review the protocol. I met him at the airport. He stepped off the plane,
after an overnight flight, wearing a dark-maroon velour suit without
a wrinkle in it. "Did you fly standing up?" I said. He was about my
age. And like Veronesi, he was flamboyant, fun loving, and handsome, with dark wavy hair, a square, rugged face, and a fetching gap-
toothed smile. The nurses went gaga over him.

He was also very smart. For a week, he sat in the module next to my lab, reviewing the pilot study, patient by patient. Eventually, he and Veronesi agreed to do the study if we paid for the trial, because the Italian government wouldn't. We even set up and paid for a clinical trials office that could support future studies with them as partners, because the Italian government wouldn't pay for that, either.

A study that we'd also piloted using a single drug—L-phenylalanine mustard, better known as L-PAM—in the postoperative period was published in *The New England Journal of Medicine* in January 1975.[2] It had been tested by Bernie Fisher, a surgeon and researcher who had forever earned the ire of fellow surgeons for challenging the notion that surgery was enough. The adjuvant CMF trial was published a year later in February 1976 by Bonadonna.

Both studies were positive, but the results of the CMF study were particularly good and made Bonadonna famous. The CMF study was the first to show a positive effect of adjuvant therapy on mortality in breast cancer.

The L-PAM study was published shortly after Betty Ford, the wife of the president, Gerald R. Ford, and Happy Rockefeller, Governor Nelson Rockefeller's wife, were diagnosed with breast cancer. I was asked to consult on both cases. Even though both women were beyond the period in which patients were started on L-PAM in the study, the drug's success raised the question of whether they could still benefit from using adjuvant treatment, and in each case, we were asked about it. We knew the study on CMF was coming out soon because we had designed CMF and paid for the study, so we recommended postoperative chemotherapy. Betty Ford went on to be treated with Fisher's L-PAM. The wife of the president couldn't take the risk of the new combination drug treatment—too many unknowns and visible side effects like hair loss for a very public person. Happy Rockefeller received no further treatment because she was operated on at Memorial Sloan Kettering, where the surgeons still thought we were nuts. Fortunately for her, her cancer did not recur.

Medicine branch studies were organized so that every year we had one or more papers to present at the cancer meetings. Within the span of five years, we'd proved we could cure advanced Hodgkin's disease with MOPP; that maintenance therapy was not needed after remission in Hodgkin's disease; and that MOPP alone was superior to radiotherapy in early-stage disease, confirming Skipper's inverse rule in humans.

We'd also shown that DLBCL was curable by chemotherapy. We called our paper on the study, published in the British journal *The Lancet* in 1975, "Advanced Diffuse Histiocytic Lymphoma, a Potentially Curable Disease: Results with Combination Chemotherapy."[3] We'd been inspired by Eric Easson and Marion Russell, who had caught my attention—and scandalized the scientific community— by using the word "cure" in the title of their paper regarding Hodgkin's disease in 1963.

We weren't exaggerating. We had cured our second cancer.

The principles we'd used to develop MOPP enabled us to devise numerous treatments, including CMF, which would become the standard of adjuvant treatment for the disease it was meant to treat, breast cancer, for the next twenty years. The face of cancer treatment was changing for good. Adjuvant chemotherapy, the use of cancer drugs coupled with surgery and/or radiotherapy, had been born.

The atmosphere on the wards was vastly different from what it had been ten years earlier, when I'd arrived at the NCI. Now our trainees felt as if they were on a mission. Morale was high. Occasionally, a young doctor realized he couldn't handle seeing patients his own age battling cancer. We usually relocated these doctors early and advised them to switch fields. Taking care of cancer patients wasn't for everybody. But if it was for you, 12 West was where you wanted to be.

We were very proud of what we were doing. The war on cancer had given us a boost, and scientific advances in the treatment of cancer were happening almost faster than we could document them. But elsewhere, the war on cancer was not proceeding as smoothly. The passage of the National Cancer Act was followed almost immediately by a misguided planning process that would lead nowhere.

After the cancer act was passed, Carl Baker became director of the

NCI. He was a likable man, always nicely dressed and polite, but he lacked a commanding presence. For most of his career, he had been an administrator. He had little firsthand knowledge about research and no clinical experience and couldn't make the connection between the lab and the clinic. What separates great doctors from mediocre doctors is the ability to integrate all the information they see in their patients, on the wards, on a day-to-day basis and understand it. Many people who are mostly administrators cannot connect what they do to clinical circumstances, because they have never been in that situation. Baker was primarily an administrator. Congress, as Mary Lasker well knew, was looking for insight into problems that affected real people. Congressmen grill enough people at hearings that competent ones can detect a fudged answer. When Baker was pushed or when he was giving testimony before Congress, his lack of confidence in his own knowledge came through. Mary Lasker spotted this immediately. He only lasted a year before being asked to step down.

In 1972, Frank Rauscher, known to everyone as Dick, replaced Baker. Rauscher was a well-known cancer virologist and a very congenial guy—a cherubic forty-one-year-old with a ready and appealing laugh. And Mary both knew him and liked him, especially in light of her conviction that viruses were a cause of cancer. In part, it had been Dick's discovery of the cancer-causing mouse virus named after him, the Rauscher leukemia virus, that led Mary to push Congress, two years later, to allocate funds for the Special Virus Cancer Program.

It was extremely controversial from the start because not many people besides Mary believed that cancer might be caused by viruses, including Ken Endicott.* And the program was despised by the NIH because to spend its largesse rapidly, the program had sidestepped the R01 grant process, copied the NCI's drug development program (the one that had brought Skipper and his crew in), and used contracts to

---

*It is now widely agreed that worldwide about a quarter of all cancers are caused by viruses, including liver and cervical cancers.

allocate its funds and support its research. Rauscher had been the head of the program since 1964, and he knew his way around the controversies. And he knew we would have to finance many of the new programs by using contracts.

But Rauscher had two major weaknesses as director. One was that he had zero clinical skills or interest in that direction. This was a problem because Congress, to whom the director of the NCI had to report four or five times a year with an update, wanted to hear about what progress was being made on the clinical front. Any such information had to be fed to Rauscher by someone with clinical experience. (Usually it was me.) What's more, the money awarded to the NCI because of clinical advances was overwhelmingly going to support basic research. We needed basic research, but we also, per the requirement of the National Cancer Act, needed to apply the results of that research to patients as quickly as possible.

Rauscher also had a well-known weakness for alcohol. Every day, he and his immediate staff, known around the NIH as "the palace guard," had a three-martini lunch at the Red Lion Inn on Wisconsin Avenue. Everyone knew that if you wanted to talk serious business, you met with Rauscher in the morning. If you wanted something from him, it was best to see him in the afternoon, when he was always more generous.

The palace guardians were mostly close poker-playing friends of his. It appeared that they thought the war on cancer was just a big source of money to use to accrue power as they handed it out to their friends.

To really effect change, the NCI had to be reorganized so that the departments of chemotherapy, radiotherapy, and surgery could work more cooperatively. This had happened, to a degree. After the act was passed, a new division had been created at the NCI—the Division of Cancer Treatment—more commonly referred to as the DCT. It was meant to be the main clearinghouse for the war on cancer, through which scientists both inside and outside the NCI advanced new therapies and incorporated all the tools we now had—basic research findings related to cancer treatment, radiation, surgery, and chemotherapy. Gordon Zubrod had been named its director.

But the DCT had one major flaw: only chemotherapy was under its domain. The other essential components—radiotherapy and surgery and related basic research—were in a separate division awkwardly called the Division of Biology and Diagnosis. The group that conducted large-scale clinical trials was in yet another division—headed by a scientist who had zero understanding of clinical-trial issues.

Zubrod needed to be in charge of all three divisions in order to set national priorities for treatment research that combined all three approaches. But he wasn't, and the three divisions didn't agree on much of anything. And there was no way Zubrod could set priorities without having final authority over all three departments and the cooperative groups. Naturally, he wanted all the treatment components under his purview, and he'd asked for that repeatedly, from each director, but to no avail. Those who ran the other divisions didn't want to lose control of their programs, and the NCI director who could have made the change didn't force them to do it. Outside the NCI, radiotherapists and surgeons were also opposed to the consolidation. They were afraid of the accumulation of authority in the hands of someone who was not one of their own.

So the DCT was the old chemotherapy program with a new name, fighting the same turf battles with radiotherapists and surgeons, who did not like the idea that chemotherapists might become as important in the treatment of cancer as they were.

This was a major failure. If we couldn't get the scientists and the doctors to cooperate with one another at the administrative level, how could we ever get them to work together on new treatments?

In the early 1970s, therapy was generally given in sequence—surgery first, followed by radiotherapy and, as a last resort, chemotherapy. There was some variation. Which therapy the patient got first in this sequence was ordained by whoever saw the patient first. If it was a surgeon, surgery was first. A radiotherapist would start with radiotherapy. When therapies were combined, which wasn't often, the individual treatments were usually given as if they were being used alone: maximum surgery, maximum radiotherapy, and maximum chemotherapy. The consequence was sometimes horrific, disfiguring toxicity.

What was needed were studies, like the ones we had done in the medicine branch with Hodgkin's disease, to answer such questions as how much of each therapy was actually necessary or if one could be substituted for another. Without central coordination of these trials, no progress could be made. The NCI was regularly asked at congressional hearings whether all of its scientists and programs were working together. The NCI said yes, of course, even though its administrators knew that wasn't true.

And then there were the groups that ran the national clinical trials—the clinical cooperative groups—which operated more like competitive sports teams. If one group made a useful observation, another group would often develop a different but similar program to call its own. Then the groups would argue about whose version was better. It was more about egos than helping patients.

Also, each group knew that when it completed a study, it had to launch a new one immediately or risk losing its share of research funds. Great ideas aren't always immediately obvious, however. Yet investigators in the cooperative groups got into the habit of starting new studies—even unnecessary ones—just to keep something going.

The cooperative groups were doing boring, repetitive, and wasteful clinical studies that didn't advance our understanding of how to deliver effective treatment, cost money, and tied up resources. And in the meantime, when good ideas arose, they were often held up until these pointless studies were completed.

The NCI needed tough new leadership to correct this state of affairs. I had great respect for Gordon Zubrod. He was a good man. He could have done it, but he was thwarted by internal politics. And no NCI director was responsive to Zubrod's frequent pleading to allow him to do what he was expected to do. It was a mess.

Meanwhile, we were facing the deadline Mary Lasker had imposed upon us. In the flurry of public relations she'd generated to push the National Cancer Act through Congress, she had spread the word that if the bill passed, we could conquer cancer by 1976, the nation's bicentennial. It would be a birthday gift to the nation. Nixon himself had repeated the promise during an address to Congress.

Everyone in the field knew it was absurd. The act was signed in late 1971, and money wasn't available until a year later. New cancer centers were not established until 1974, and then only a few. It took these centers three to five years to recruit scientists, construct buildings, and set up laboratories. There was no chance of the National Cancer Act having any measurable impact by 1976. I don't think Mary believed it was possible, either. She merely thought it was a necessary tactic to get the act passed.

But the congressmen and senators who had helped pass the act did not know this, nor did the general public. Given the promises that had been made, we were all bracing for the firestorm that would come when 1976 arrived and we did not have "a" cure. Meanwhile, Mary never eased up on the pressure she put on Congress for funding. And her attention to detail was impressive.

When she visited Washington, she stayed at Deeda Blair's stately home on Foxhall Road, where she and Deeda had a continuous run of dinner parties and luncheons. I attended many of them. I quickly noticed that the seating arrangements were carefully drawn. People like me were always seated next to someone we might be able to influence. And after dinner, Deeda would always get up and ask one of the famous scientists present to give "spontaneous remarks about the work they were doing." These after-dinner talks, of course, had been carefully arranged to conform to Mary's plans. I know because I spoke at a number of these dinners and was "coached," just to be sure I planned to say the right things. You could count on seeing members of Congress and other influential people in the administration at the dinner tables.

She did the same thing at the luncheons for the awarding of the Lasker prizes each year held in the St. Regis hotel roof ballroom and social events at her town house on Beekman Place in Manhattan. I always found myself seated next to a reporter or opinion leader who might gather some positive information from me for a future story.

And the luncheons at Deeda's house were something else again. One particularly sticks in my mind. One morning, I was called by Deeda Blair, asking me to come to lunch. I had meetings and clinics to attend that day, so I declined. A sense of urgency entered Deeda's voice, and she said it was critical and that Mary would very much appreciate it if I would drop everything and come to lunch. Reluctantly, I had my secretary rearrange my schedule. I arrived at Deeda's house a little late and saw a big black government sedan in the circular driveway and was introduced, as we sat down, to a Mr. Featherstone Reid. Lunch went as usual with nice food and conversation, with Mary turning to me frequently and saying, "Vince, why don't you tell Featherstone about all the marvelous advances we are making." I did, and after an hour and a half Mr. Reid excused himself, saying he had to return to Congress, and left.

Mary took her coffee to the couch in Deeda's living room and sat down. By now, I was very curious about why Mr. Reid was so important, so I sat next to her and said, "Mary, who is Featherstone Reid?" She looked at me with a straight face and said, "He is Maggie's driver." Maggie was the nickname for Warren Magnuson, a senator and chair of the Senate Appropriations Committee, Mary's old friend. My frustration at being called away from my work to have lunch with "Maggie's driver" broke through, and I started to object. Mary stopped me with an upraised hand and said, "Vince, he drives Maggie to work every morning and after that he drives Mrs. Maggie shopping all day. And Mrs. Maggie is the last person to put her head on the pillow next to Maggie each night."

I must admit I was amused. Poor Warren Magnuson, who was her good friend anyhow, was being surrounded by people, including his driver, who would bombard him day and night with positive news supporting Mary's requests for funds. He didn't stand a chance. I chuckled all the way back to my office.

Her visits to congressmen and senators were also quite an experience. Quinn told me she would even visit those he said were hostile on the chance she could charm them into changing their minds. Once we visited a congressman from Florida who Quinn had said was a no go for increases in the NCI budget. And he was. He kept us waiting for forty-five minutes, unheard of for Mary in my experience. It was good for me because at times like these, Mary would tell me more stories about how she got things done. But I could see the smoke coming out of her ears while we waited. And when we went in, he sat there with a glaze over his eyes, clearly sending a message that he was not impressed by Mary. He would be subjected to a Soloman Garb letter-writing campaign. There were not many like that, though.

She was usually received with gusto. More like it were her visits to see Senator Hubert Humphrey. They were good friends, and she took me along on several visits. The first time we went right in, and they hugged and kissed and made small talk for about five minutes before Mary got around to introducing me.* Before we went in, Mary had said to me, "I'm going to ask him for a $200 million increase over the president's budget." Panicked, I told her there was no way I could think of things to justify that kind of an increase. She gave me an angry look because she hated people to tell her they couldn't spend money. She just told me to be enthusiastic and not to worry about it because she usually only got half of what she asked for anyhow.

Sure enough, when we were through extolling the virtues of cancer research, she asked him to add $200 million to the NCI appropriation. He protested the amount and said he would put a request in for

---

*Her coldness occasionally surprised me, too. In the late 1970s, when Hubert Humphrey was quite ill with metastatic bladder cancer and I was the consultant on his case, she would pump me for information. Because his case was quite public and I knew they were friends, I told her that he was not likely to be around much longer. At one point, after a huggy-kissy visit to the office of the now-quite-frail Humphrey, she sat me down and said, "You know, Vince, we have to prepare for this. Hubert's death will get us a lot of publicity, and we can get more money added to the budget." She was right.

$100 million and picked up the phone and instructed his staff to do so on the spot. And we got an extra $100 million that year, when all was said and done. My conscience was assuaged when I calculated that about $5 million had gone into the clinical studies I had discussed as candidates for the $200 million and $95 million went into our basic research program. Mary was shrewd and knew it worked out this way.

One day in 1974, after three years of struggling and failing to bring the Division of Cancer Treatment into line, Zubrod walked into Rauscher's office and quit. He knew he couldn't do the job that needed to be done without the proper organizational structure, and he'd had it.

Shortly afterward, Dick Rauscher called me into his office. He motioned for me to sit in one of two black leather armchairs in the corner, near the big windows facing north, and he took the other. We made small talk as we watched a rainstorm march toward us. I didn't know why I was there—until Rauscher decided it was time to tell me.

"Vince," he said, "I want you to replace Gordon Zubrod." I almost fell off that armchair.

I fumbled around a bit, pointing out all the things he already knew: that I would be a surprise choice; that I would be promoted over all of the division's associate directors, which was bound to make them unhappy. I mentioned that I would need to ask for some changes. I knew exactly why Zubrod had left, and I didn't blame him. He was a visionary who wasn't being allowed to do his work. "I can't take the job unless the treatment division becomes a real treatment division," I said. "All of the intramural and extramural treatment programs need to be moved under my direction."

He sat there looking at me for so long I thought he hadn't heard me. I could see he was struggling with my response, which, admittedly, had been cheeky. I was being offered one of the most powerful cancer treatment jobs in the world, and already I was making demands. But I knew that it couldn't be done without the changes I'd requested. To take responsibility without the requisite authority would be folly.

He ran his hand through his hair, rubbed his nose, gazed out the window, and then twisted around in his seat, and looked across the room as if someone would materialize to help him deal with this issue. After a while, he turned and looked at me, heaved a big sigh, laughed his jolly laugh, and said, "Okay, Vince, I'll do it, but it will raise holy hell with the other division directors."

Now I was in the hot seat. I stared back at him, at an unusual loss for words. I was among those who'd been skeptical about the promises of the National Cancer Act. But I'd come to believe that Mary Lasker's vision wasn't wrong or illogical. Just overly ambitious. As chief of medicine, I'd seen a lot and had ideas about how to change things in the treatment division, and I didn't need a long period of indoctrination to begin to move.

I had often fantasized about the proper organization of the Division of Cancer Treatment. I would have to take over the functions of the clinical director, then headed by a doctor with little clinical experience. I also thought we needed an external advisory board that could review the budgets and research programs of all of the branches that would be under my control. The NIH scrutinized every grant given to universities that conducted research outside the NIH. But it was irritating to those scientists that they never saw what we were doing on the inside. The advisory board would resolve that and create a system of accountability. I also knew that this wouldn't sit well with the rest of the NCI or the NIH, which preferred to be opaque to outsiders.

We also needed to reevaluate the old drug-screening process that had been in place since I arrived at the NCI in 1963. Since the drug-screening program began, we'd relied on the L1210 leukemia cells grown in CDF1 mice. It had been a good way to start, and it helped pave the way in leukemia. But we had outgrown it. People had lost confidence in it as an effective way to identify new cancer drugs. How could screening chemicals for their effects against one mouse leukemia possibly reflect what would happen against many different kinds of human cancers, they said. I had studied the way L1210 grew and knew it did not grow the way common solid cancers grew in humans. We needed a model that used transplanted bits of human tumors in mice engineered to allow them to grow. It was time for a change. But the drug-screening program was built on cronyism. People had spent their entire careers doing research around the L1210 system. Companies existed solely to produce the two million CDF1 mice used each year to grow L1210, and other companies existed to screen the forty thousand new chemicals evaluated each year for effectiveness against cancer. It was an industry in itself. The many ben-eficiaries of this system were not inclined to support new programs that might put their funding at risk. The drug-screening program cost $100 million a year. It wouldn't be easy to change it.

And most important of all, we needed to support new and bright researchers because the future of cancer rested on them. My hope was to link both intramural research (research taking place at the NCI) and extramural research (NCI-supported research taking place at uni-versities) in cancer treatment in ways that would accelerate progress.

There were many bright people who were prominent critics of our drug development program. One was the great basic scientist Charlie Heidelberger, the discoverer of the cancer drug 5-fluorouracil, the first real targeted therapy. His studies had shown that cancers took up one of the chemical components of RNA, uracil, more avidly than normal tissue did. He had cleverly designed the drug with a fluorine atom attached to it that looked a lot like uracil. When it was taken up by cancer cells, it irreversibly inhibited an enzyme vital to DNA synthesis, thymidylate synthase. I wanted him on the board. And the other critics, too. They needed to see how we spent our money. And we needed their ideas, and their critiques, to make sure we were doing our best and were not too attached to approaches that weren't working. All researchers can use another pair of eyes—or a dozen pairs—to make sure they stay on the right track.

As part of the transfer of the cooperative group program to DCT, we needed to bring in the controversial National Surgical Adjuvant Breast Project, or NSABP. The NSABP was run by Bernie Fisher, the breast surgeon, who had dared to challenge the status quo by researching and ultimately supporting the use of adjuvant therapy for breast cancer—and had also been castigated for it.

The Colorado physician Dr. Juan del Regato, one of the founding fathers of radiotherapy and a member of the National Advisory Cancer Council, had been incensed over Fisher's studies showing that postoperative radiotherapy didn't work for breast cancer and, in fact, only added to the morbidity of treatment. Del Regato persuaded the chair of the NACC, Dr. Sidney Farber, and other members of the board to cut off all funds used for follow-up of NSABP patients, essentially killing the program. If you can't follow patients, you can't document your results. It was a vindictive maneuver, done behind closed doors to protect his specialty—to hell with the patients.

The NSABP was now in the hole for about $350,000 as a result of the action of the National Advisory Cancer Council. The DCT would have to take on the debt. But it was by far one of the most productive groups in my opinion. It had to be saved.

Moving from chief of medicine to director of the DCT would take me away from the day-to-day contact with patients, whom I loved treating. I wasn't just administering state-of-the-art cancer medicine; I was creating it. That's a rare opportunity for a doctor. And it was more than gratifying to see these patients come back year after year bubbling with life. At the time, I was still following a leukemia patient I had treated when I was a clinical associate and she was in her early teens. Ten years later, she had gone to college, married, and had a child, whom she proudly brought to the clinic to show me. It brought me to tears, and I don't cry easily.

Not all stories had happy endings, but it was still a privilege to be a part of them. I had one patient, a teenage boy, whom we were treating for acute leukemia. His mother, a single parent, had been a constant presence in the hospital. A year before Phil was due to graduate from high school, she developed metastatic breast cancer. It seemed, ironically, that he would survive and she would not. The one thing she wanted was to see him graduate from high school. By the time of graduation, she was too weak to go on her own steam. So I arranged for an ambulance to take her to the graduation, which was outdoors, and park on the hill. She watched from a stretcher. She died shortly afterward. And Phil eventually relapsed, too. But they meant something, these moments. They not only taught you what it means to be a doctor, and a human being, but gave you opportunities to step up and be one.

"Can I have some time to think about it?" I asked Rauscher. He nodded his assent and rose from his chair. The meeting was over. During this time, I often thought of Freireich, one of the people who had instructed and inspired me, taught me, and made my career possible. Freireich had once likened working with the young leukemia patients at the NIH to the stories that appear fleetingly, in newspapers or on the nightly news, in which a child has fallen off a dock and a random guy who can't swim feels compelled to jump in and grab the kid and manages to save him.

Doctors on the cancer wards had the same choice, he said. You could jump in, despite dubious odds, or you could sit by and say it'll never work and let the child die. Freireich had long since made up his mind about the right course of action. "You become involved," he said. "There's no other option. How could I let kids die without doing what I think can be done?"

Trying your best for a patient and, hopefully, saving him or her turns you into an optimist, he said. For him, optimism had become a sort of evangelism. He knew, he said, that every patient he saw would somehow get something better than the one before, and he was determined to make that happen. Seeing what I had seen, both as Freireich's student and then in my own work with Hodgkin's, I had become an optimist, too.

A month after Rauscher offered me the job, I told him I'd take it.

As I'd predicted, it wasn't popular news. When the word got around, the people I'd been promoted over threatened to quit. Word of the demands I'd made with regard to the DCT stirred up a hornet's nest, too. People didn't bother taking their complaints to Rauscher. They thought they'd been betrayed by him. They went right to Benno Schmidt, the head of the President's Cancer Panel. If he submitted to the pressure and told Rauscher to find someone else, I was cooked.

The President's Cancer Panel was set up as part of the National Cancer Act. It consisted of three members, a layperson who chaired it, a basic scientist, and a clinician. The panel had oversight responsibility for the entire NCI, including the operation of the newly created National Cancer Advisory Board, or NCAB. The panel was appointed by the president and reported directly to him.

The NCAB was also appointed by the president and was made up of twenty-two members, six of them laypeople. This had been the great compromise to keep the NCI in the NIH and satisfy Mary Lasker that the program would have the freedom to operate independently. Mary, always suspicious of NIH leadership, wanted to bypass it and most especially arrange things so that laypeople were involved, to be sure money was spent on programs for people—not just programs to keep researchers employed.

By law, the cancer panel met twelve times a year. The NCI director prepared a budget and submitted it directly to the president through the cancer panel, bypassing the NIH budget office and the Department of Health and Human Services, which technically had oversight of it. It forevermore became known as the bypass budget.

Benno Schmidt had been President Nixon's choice to head the new panel. And Schmidt bypassed everybody. After each panel meeting, he got in a limo and went to see Nixon or, at a very minimum, Bob Haldeman, his chief of staff, to discuss the NCI's need for resources. It was protocol for the director of the NCI and the chair of the board to lead the NCAB meetings. But Carl Baker, and the other directors who followed, had all ceded control to Schmidt.

Schmidt was the managing partner of the venture capital firm

J. H. Whitney and chair of the board of managers of the Memorial Sloan Kettering Cancer Center. He was the guy credited with coining the phrase "venture capital." Having an overseer function at Memorial meant he was no stranger to medical intrigue, either.

Because I was chief of medicine when the act was passed, I was senior enough to sit in on board and panel meetings, and I got to watch Schmidt in action.

He was well over six feet tall, square shouldered, and handsome. He had bushy white eyebrows and a full head of dark-brown hair with a shock of white in the front and over his temples. Without fail, he wore a dark blue suit, stood straight as an arrow with his shoulders back, and walked with a confident stride, like John Wayne without the hitch in his step. He had a deep, gravelly voice with a thick Texas drawl that I took to imitating for my colleagues back at the medicine branch.

He was one of the few laypeople I knew who could dissect complicated medical problems faster than most physicians and scientists. Once, I'd seen the head of the cancer control program try to justify a flawed mammography program that was costing millions of dollars a year. I knew it was problematic, but it was presented as God's gift to women. Most of the NCAB fell for it. Schmidt didn't. And he didn't just express his concern; he coolly and justifiably destroyed the logic that was presented. The program was stopped, and the director was perpetually terrified of him thereafter. You didn't present garbage to Schmidt and expect it to go unnoticed.

He exuded confidence and was fearless in dealing with unruly, arrogant board members.

Jim Watson, of double helix fame, had been appointed to the NCAB because he was a brilliant scientist. But he also hated the concept of the war on cancer and was purposefully rude at board meetings to show his contempt. The board chair couldn't control him. Watson was, after all, a Nobel laureate. He liked to lean back and put his feet up on the table and read *The New York Times*, lowering the paper only to interject a derogatory comment here and there. Schmidt patiently waited for the board chair to say something, but he didn't. On one occasion, when the board was discussing the newly formed Cancer Centers Program, Watson lowered the paper and said, "This is a pile of shit."

Benno asked for the floor and said, "I have the budget of the centers program here." He then noted that one of the largest grants went to "Dr. Watson at Cold Spring Harbor." "Are you part of the pile of shit, Dr. Watson?" A stunned Jim Watson put the paper and his feet down and remained silent. His bluff had been called. Then Schmidt got in his limo and went to the White House and asked that a disruptive Jim Watson be removed from the board. Watson's six-year appointment was terminated after two years. You didn't want to mess with Benno Schmidt, even if you had a Nobel Prize. In 2009, Jim wrote an editorial in *The New York Times* claiming that he had been booted because "the NCI went clinical," which wasn't even close to being true.[4] Then and now, about 85 percent of the NCI's budget went to supporting basic research.

When Schmidt contacted me and told me he wanted to hear why I thought the NCI needed to be restructured, I was rattled. We met in Rauscher's office. He listened intently, occasionally raising his bushy white eyebrows when I explained how some of the directors were operating out of selfish reasons. He was surprised, I think, that I was being so frank. But my guess is he already suspected what was going on.

To my relief, he immediately saw the logic. I wasn't even finished with my presentation when he got up from his chair and began to walk around the room while he talked. "Vince," he said, in his gravelly voice, "I think I know how to fix this." We then spent the better part of an hour strategizing over how to quell the revolt. Schmidt's solution was a series of dinners to be held over the next few weeks, first with disaffected senior staff I'd suddenly outranked, then with the heads of the departments to be transferred. The final obstacle was meeting with the chairs of the cooperative groups.* He wanted to hear directly from them why they objected to what I'd proposed.

Over the course of the next several weeks, Schmidt took us to good restaurants in nearby Washington, D.C. Schmidt, who was rumored to be worth about $500 million, paid the tabs himself. He and I usually traveled to the restaurants together in his rented Mercedes limo. A few times, we took taxis when he hadn't been able to schedule a car service. Like a lot of rich people, Schmidt didn't carry cash with him, so when this happened, I, who made about $25,000 a year, ended up paying the cab fares out of my own pocket.

The compensation was that the dinners worked brilliantly. Schmidt wasn't impressed with the usual self-serving, turf-protecting arguments he'd heard. I didn't have to say much. I could see that even the people making their cases were uncomfortable.

Schmidt asked all the people we met with what they wanted of me. The new chief of surgery, Steve Rosenberg, just wanted to be left alone to do his research. The chief of radiotherapy, Ralph Johnson, with whom Moxley and I had wrestled over MOMP, just wanted me to go away. All ten cooperative group chairs knew that I wasn't thrilled with what they'd been doing. They wanted a guarantee that I wouldn't abolish them, but that wasn't my plan. We needed the clinical trials program. But they needed to be reorganized and, in some cases, consolidated to focus their studies on national protocols addressing important questions. Busywork studies had to stop. Cross-group collaboration had to start.

---

*The division directors who had resisted the change when Zubrod asked for it were Dr. Nathaniel Berlin and Dr. Thomas King. Both eventually left. The two associate directors I leapfrogged were Paul Carbone and Steve Carter. Paul left for the University of Wisconsin, and Steve became my deputy and taught me a lot about opera. The branch chiefs were Dr. Ralph Johnson, chief of radiotherapy; Dr. Steve Rosenberg, chief of surgery; and Dr. Arthur Levine, chief of pediatrics. Dr. Johnson left to set up a cancer center in Florida. Dr. Rosenberg went on to a brilliant career developing immunotherapy for cancer at the NCI. Dr. Levine eventually left for a career in academic administration at the University of Pittsburgh.

The upshot was that two people I'd stepped over for the job left, and the others had to back down. I was in. I was in charge of managing the country's treatment effort and distributing most of the resources available for research and development for cancer treatment. And for the first time, the DCT was actually a real treatment division.

I was ready.

The new organization had an immediate effect on the design of new trials. With money available, the National Surgical Adjuvant Breast Project led the way, using lab-based scientific logic in reducing the use of surgery and radiotherapy and adding adjuvant chemotherapy for the treatment of breast cancer. And the other groups followed.

As the results from studies rolled in, the findings suggested that if you treated the primary tumor and, at the same time, the cells that had escaped with chemotherapy, you could prevent recurrences. This meant that surgery and radiation didn't necessarily need to go wide or deep for better effect.

A remarkable change began to take hold in the field of cancer treatment. Surgeons began to shape their operations around the availability of these other treatments; radiotherapists did the same. You didn't need to do the classic "cancer operation" if the drugs were going to take care of any escaped cells anyhow.

Because they no longer needed to focus on the size of the operation, surgeons refined their techniques. Surgery for colorectal cancer, for instance, had once involved removing the entire colon, which required the patient to use a colostomy bag for the rest of his life. Now, thanks to improved surgical technique, colostomies were often not necessary.

Limbs were being spared. Instead of going so far as to disarticulate a hip for a tumor in a leg bone, the tumors were removed and the bone replaced by a prosthesis.

Radiation treatment to the primary site and chemotherapy took care of the escaped cells here, too. In head and neck cancers, radiotherapy took a lead role, and less radical procedures are now used. The commando operation became a thing of the past.

But these advances weren't enough to keep the promise that Mary had made. As we knew, the bicentennial celebration would come and go without a cure for cancer. And the predictable articles on the "failed" war on cancer started to appear in the mainstream press. "U.S. Cancer Program Termed 'Sham,'" screamed a headline in March 1975 in *The Boston Globe*.[5] "Dissent Against the War on Cancer," read the headline of an editorial in April 1975, which said that high-level critics of America's war on cancer were proliferating.[6] "War on Cancer Stirs a Political Backlash," according to *The New York Times* in May 1975,[7] while in the same year "False Front in War on Cancer" ran in the *Chicago Tribune*.[8]

The problem was twofold: These new approaches had yet to be widely implemented outside the NCI and certainly not enough to affect national mortality statistics. And the members of the press were still smarting that they'd been duped by Mary Lasker into believing we could eradicate cancer in a matter of years.

It also depended on how you defined success. For the angry critics, unless you cured *all* cancer, the war on cancer was a failure. But the reality was that we were just getting started. The laboratory research programs that would define the future of cancer biology, prevention, diagnosis, and treatment had just gotten under way. But the articles decrying the failed war on cancer would become perennial in the mainstream media.

The leadership for the NCI was still shaky. In mid-1977, Dick Rauscher resigned. He was replaced by Arthur Upton, a pathologist whose research interests were in radiobiology. Upton was a low-key, academic type with no particular belief in the war on cancer. And he hated the spotlight. He told me that each time he testified before Congress, he died a thousand deaths. He loathed it and always took me with him, and he usually turned the testimony over to me. I think members of Congress came to believe I was the NCI director. By January 1980, he was done.

When he stepped down, a search committee chaired by Benno Schmidt recommended me to President Carter as the NCI's new director. The job was offered, and I accepted, though it was not an easy time for me. Between 1972 and 1980, I had been quietly fighting a personal battle that, while it did not directly have to do with cancer, did affect my commitment to the National Cancer Act's mandate to help foster translation from the labs to the bedside.

In September 1972, while sitting down for dinner, I'd glanced at my nine-year-old son's legs. Ted's bruises would have made any oncologist's heart stop. People with a low platelet count are susceptible to a very specific type of bruising. When their platelet counts are somewhat low, the bruises appear like a scattering of blue pinpoints. When their counts are very low, the bruises are large, purple, and ugly, as if they've been left by a baseball bat. Ted's were of this variety.

In someone his age, such bruises most likely meant leukemia.

The next day, I'd brought him to work so I could get a platelet count on him. A normal count is more than 150,000. Ted's was 3,000. He had the test my patients dreaded most, a bone marrow biopsy. And soon, we knew. It was not leukemia. It was worse. Aplastic anemia is an extremely rare disease in which the marrow stops producing red and white blood cells and platelets.

As in leukemia, patients with aplastic anemia were at risk of bleeding to death or dying from infection. But because it was so rare—the disease equivalent of getting struck by lightning—there had never been an impetus to search for a cure, nor any research funds to support such a search. As a result, there was nothing. In 20 percent of patients, the bone marrow spontaneously started working again within a year. The rest died within that time frame.

Ted's counts put him in the category of patients with the worst prognosis. Our only option was to give him transfusions of platelets and red blood cells as a temporary fix and wait to see if his bone marrow started working again. Plan B—the idea of the doctor I'd consulted with at the NCI—had been to put him in one of the sterile rooms Freireich had invented years earlier to protect leukemia patients from infection and that he'd insisted we use while we were developing MOMP.

Plan A worked for two weeks. But then Ted spiked a fever, and option B went into effect. We thought it would be just to stabilize and support him during the agonizing wait to see if his bone marrow would start working again. But something unexpected happened. His bone marrow did not start again, but the sterile environment protected him from germs, and the transfusions kept him going. In the room, he could live.

For the next eight years, I'd spend my days on 12 West, working on behalf of cancer patients, always aware that Ted was one floor above me, in his sterile room on 13 East. Meanwhile, I scoured medical journals and enlisted the opinion of any scientists or clinicians who'd ever encountered aplastic anemia, looking for anything that might help him.

We'd tried treating Ted with a series of androgens, male hormones, because they'd been shown to enhance blood cell production in some studies. They'd helped for a time, but the effect hadn't lasted. I'd seen a report about elevated white blood cell counts in patients with manic depression who took lithium to control their symptoms. The drug, somehow, appeared to stimulate the bone marrow. We tried that, too. Ted's white cell count had risen but fallen again.

We'd tried crude colony-stimulating factors, proteins that signal stem cells in the marrow to proliferate. But they'd been too new, too unrefined, and they hadn't worked. There was a theory that aplastic anemia was an autoimmune disease that occurred when the body's own T cells attacked the marrow. We'd tried giving Ted an anti-lymphocyte serum (T cells are lymphocytes). But it had only made him sicker. We'd looked into the then-new approach of bone marrow transplant, but Ted's sister, the most likely donor, was not a match, and we'd not been able to find another.

Meanwhile, we'd kept him stable with transfusions. But we knew that their effectiveness could not last and that the side effects of the blood transfusions would eventually become a problem.

Red blood cells carry iron molecules that help bind oxygen to them, which they then carry to our organs. Red cells have a finite life span;

when they die, they release their iron. Normally, the body reuses it for the other red cells the marrow produces. But because Ted wasn't producing any other red cells, the iron from his transfusions had no place to go. Eventually, we knew that it would encrust his heart, damaging the muscle and the electrical conduction system that kept it beating, causing his heart to fail.

For eight years, we'd desperately tried to find something to help him before that happened. But on May 27, 1980, we lost the battle.

Why do I tell you this story? Because, though I had certainly been committed to my patients and their families and empathized with their struggles and their losses, I had not, until that day at the dinner table in 1972, been one of them. I had not known exactly what it was like to hope against hope that something would come out of the lab soon enough to help someone you loved. I had learned what it meant to be on the other side in the most shattering way possible.

Cancer had once been where aplastic anemia was. Not rare, but ignored, the realm of a handful of doctors with scant resources and few advances flowing from the lab. It had resources now, but the effort for a cure was moving more slowly than it had to. I believed in what Mary Lasker had started, and I understood the mission of the National Cancer Act. I wanted to see what would happen if we used all the resources we had. It was time to truly put it into action.

On a warm day in July 1980, in the plush new auditorium of the National Library of Medicine, I placed my hand on the worn Bible that Mary Kay had inherited from her grandmother and was sworn in as director of the National Cancer Institute. I was now in control of the most powerful institute for cancer research in the world.

7

When I walked into my new office on my first day, it smelled like wet paint. It wasn't from the walls, my secretary explained. It was from Arthur Upton's portrait. According to tradition, a photograph was taken of each director when he left office. All the portraits hung in the grand hall on the eleventh floor of the cancer center. But because Upton's wife was an artist, she'd insisted on painting his. She'd dropped it off in the office, still wet, on an easel. Someone had moved it to the conference room down the hall, but it had left the scent of fresh paint behind.

I dropped my briefcase and went to the conference room to check it out. I was startled when I lifted the canvas drop cloth. Arthur's image was distorted; he had a deer-in-the-headlights look on his face. My initial thought was that either his wife was a terrible artist or she didn't like him very much. My second thought was that maybe this was what running the National Cancer Institute had done to him. Whatever the explanation, the portrait wasn't very flattering. I wanted to put it in storage rather than hang it. But I wasn't prepared to take on Arthur's wife, should she stop by to admire it. As soon as it was dry, it went up on the wall with the other images of past directors.

I had more important battles to fight. This time, I wouldn't be doing verbal battle with a reluctant doctor over whether to use the full dose of a drug. Most of my battles would be political. I would be wearing a suit every day instead of a lab coat. And though I'd been testifying in front of Congress, as a favor, on behalf of former directors, this time the responsibility was all mine. I was here to reform the NCI and make it fit the vision of the National Cancer Act.

By 1980, the NCI's budget was approaching $1 billion. But we were in the hot seat. Scientists in other fields hated the institute because they thought it was the beneficiary of unwarranted largesse—the result of an overblown PR campaign led by a socialite who didn't understand science. They saw the NCI's large budget as a threat to their own fields. The NCI's money would have to come from somewhere, and they didn't want it to come from them. Many cancer researchers were upset, too. They resented the cure-on-demand nature of the war on cancer: we give you the money, and you give us the cure. Scientists generally preferred to turn that around: The money, they believed, should follow the discoveries. We'll show you an important finding, and you give us the money to expand our work on it.

The rest of the NIH wasn't pleased, either. They didn't like the war on cancer, because the NCI, which had once been under the NIH umbrella, now had unique powers that circumvented the NIH's authority—namely, its own budget; a director appointed by and reporting directly to the president himself; a board and a presidentially appointed cancer panel. And then there were the ever-suspicious journalists who, when the deadline for a promised cure had passed, continually looked for evidence of bungling and cover-ups.

The truth was, we were making progress. But money—the instrument of our successes—had also created new impediments. And as usual, most fell squarely in the realm of human nature. The government's financial investment in the war on cancer had turned the

National Cancer Institute into a miniversion of the Pentagon, riddled
with fiefdoms, favoritism, and decision makers intoxicated with the
power that comes from having large sums of money to distribute.

Changing the NCI into a tough, well-managed institution—with
a silhouette resembling what was described in the cancer act—that
could lead the war on cancer wasn't going to be easy. But I knew
what to do. I was probably one of the few scientists (or legislators, for
that matter) who had actually read the National Cancer Act, which
launched the war on cancer. And thanks to many hours spent with
Mary Lasker, I understood the vision that had created it. We needed
to change the NCI dramatically if it was to fulfill its mandate "to
support research, and the application of the results of research, to reduce the incidence, morbidity and mortality from cancer." I didn't
think the act was the result of a naive PR campaign. I thought Mary's
vision was achievable. I was determined to get the war on cancer back
on track, and I was willing to take risks to get there.

My first problem, however, was not the rather exalted question of
how to get the war on cancer on track but how to cope with the staff
I'd inherited from former directors, including the "palace guard," who
formed a formidable barrier around the director. As things stood,
anyone who wanted to talk to me had to go through them.

Many of them had started their careers elsewhere in the institute,
and their loyalty was to other departments. They wanted to protect
their friends from any changes a new director might have in mind.
Sometimes, without the director's knowledge, they wielded his power
in his absence. I'd encountered all of the members of the guard over
the years, and I was wary of them.

One of the most audacious was Phoebe, the previous director's
longtime secretary. It was well beyond the time when anyone at the
NCI, much less in the director's office, should have been seen smoking. But Phoebe didn't see it that way. Thanks to her, her ivory cigarette holder, and her pack-a-day habit, my office was always full of
smoke. And when we sat down to discuss my daily routine, she told

me never to make my own calls. "I do that," she explained, "so I can listen in on all of the director's calls and record them or take notes."

I was stunned. Phoebe was the J. Edgar Hoover of the cancer institute—listening in on everyone and, I soon realized, using what she learned to dole out information to people outside the office. The other members of the guard, I soon realized, were similarly exchanging information and wielding power. I replaced most of them, including Phoebe.

Eight months into my job, I faced my first political crisis. Ronald Reagan had won the presidential election, and I was a Jimmy Carter appointee. The new head of personnel in the White House, Pendleton James, had let it be known that as far as he was concerned, an empty chair was better than any Carter appointee. That didn't bode well for Don Fredrickson, the NIH director, or me. Fredrickson and I were the only two presidential appointments at the NIH. Having the director appointed by the president was considered a plus for any NIH program, because it gave the person in that position high visibility. But this was the downside. Presidential appointees served at the whim of the president and his staff, no matter how good they were.

As a matter of form, we had both tendered our resignations to the president, although we hoped they wouldn't be accepted. Don and I met once a week to share information about where our appointments stood. It was like waiting in line for your turn at the guillotine. Week after week, one resignation of a Carter appointee after another was accepted. Soon only Don and I were left.

Then I got a call from Elizabeth Dole. Over the years, I had helped her and her husband, Senator Robert Dole, when a family member or a friend had developed cancer. Elizabeth, now highly placed in the Reagan administration, told me that she was taking an interest in my appointment and tracking its progress. I had already been asked my political affiliation, and I told them it was Republican. Now I was asked to prove it. Mary Kay hustled to track down any documentation of donations I'd made to the Republican Party. Still I waited.

Finally, I got word that I'd been reappointed by President Reagan. Two weeks later, Don Fredrickson, who was a registered Democrat, got his news: he officially announced his resignation. He was replaced by James Wyngaarden, a former chief of medicine at Duke University School of Medicine and a rather famous name in the field with two slightly ominous nicknames: the Velvet Stiletto and Gentleman Jim. It was rumored that Wyngaarden didn't like the NCI, and we feared that he would make life very difficult for us.

Soon after my appointment and these other appointments were settled, another crisis emerged. I got word that *The Washington Post* would be publishing a series of articles attacking the war on cancer, to be written by two well-known investigative reporters, Ted Gup and Jonathan Neumann.

Their series was about what they characterized as a misguided attempt to develop anticancer drugs.[1] Reading their articles, I didn't get the impression that they knew much about science and medicine. One article led with the story of an eight-year-old girl, a cancer patient who, they alleged, had died as a result of an experimental drug derived from the dye in the ink used in ballpoint pens. While the drug in question had initially been developed as an ink because of its color, it had been found to have antitumor activity, and that's why it was being tested. In fact, many chemotherapy drugs are colored in solution. (Adriamycin, for example, a drug used in many combinations, is red, which is one reason patients call it "the red devil." Epirubicin is orange-red. Daunorubicin is pink in acid solution but turns purple to blue if the PH is basic.) The chemical structure of many such compounds contains benzene rings, hexagonal arrangements of carbon atoms that, in various circumstances, create color. This is a quality they share with many other chemicals, such as inks. But saying this makes them the same is like saying dogs and humans are the same because both they and we have legs. By drawing this association, as they had, in the first lines of the story, the writers had effectively put chemotherapy in the same category as snake oil.

In another article, cancer patients were described as living in "a world of disappointment and poor therapeutic results." In another, the story of a man who died of an apparent overdose of one of the drugs under study was used to portray experimental drug trials as hopeless quagmires that lured desperate cancer patients to further misery, and implied that hospitals—including prestigious ones—were not honest with patients about what they were entering into.

Again and again, patients were described as hopeless and hapless victims of mercenary doctors who were administering useless drugs without any sense of the damage they were doing. The articles were searing and deliberately misleading, among the worst examples of medical reporting I had ever seen. And it was clear to me that the reporters were being manipulated by sources from within the NIH, perhaps by some of the people I'd angered while trying to reform the cancer institute.

The articles put me in Capitol Hill's crosshairs. Some newly elected Republican senators, led by Paula Hawkins of Florida, now a member of the Senate Committee on Labor and Human Resources, decided to hold hearings on the cancer drug development program. She knew I was originally a Carter appointee. And the purpose of the hearings seemed to be to discredit me and force my resignation. Senator Orrin Hatch had assumed the chair of the committee. Ted Kennedy was the minority leader.

Senator Paula Hawkins led the hearings; Hatch and Kennedy looked on. Hawkins was a sight. She was heavily made up, with an enormous bouffant, and dressed as if she were going out on the town. It was a look that would forever earn her the nickname Betty Boop among my friends and co-workers, who watched the whole thing on C-SPAN. Hawkins was known for being utterly dependent upon her staff. She would read a statement off a piece of paper that made some kind of scandalous accusation; when I responded, she would have no idea how to answer until a staff member wrote out a reply and handed it to her, while I sat silently, waiting. I realized fairly quickly that all I had to do was answer questions and be polite. She was doing a great job of discrediting herself. When my friends and co-workers saw my polite, passive behavior (decidedly out of character) on C-SPAN, they called me up and said they were surprised and disappointed that I didn't get angry. "Where was the Vince DeVita we know?" they asked. But I'd realized there was nothing to be gained getting angry with a member of Congress during hearings. And I had bigger problems to handle than Betty Boop.

It soon became clear to me that Ted Kennedy was out to use the hearings to discredit me. I knew Kennedy pretty well because of my interactions with the FDA when I was the NCI's director of cancer treatment. Kennedy was close to the FDA and was often annoyed when I attacked the agency in public, as I often did, for being too slow and inefficient in approving new cancer drugs. I knew this because he had invited me to his office on occasion and said so.

You might think that given that his son Ted junior had had cancer and survived, years earlier, and that I was one of the doctors involved in his case, we'd be on the same side. But that wasn't the case. While many saw him as a noble statesman, my experience with him thus far had not reflected that. In my experience, despite what he'd been through with his son, he was willing to play political games with cancer.

I was accompanied by Ed Brandt, the assistant secretary for health, to the hearings every day. He was a soft-spoken Oklahoman who was a nice guy and sympathetic to my situation. While Brandt did everything he could to help, Kennedy did everything possible to discredit me with the committee chair, Orrin Hatch. Before the hearings started each day, and in full view of Hatch and Hawkins, Kennedy made a practice of coming over to the witness table, all smiles, and putting his arm around me, essentially marking me as the enemy. I knew him, but as you may surmise from my earlier comments, we were far from close friends or even collegial allies. Yet to anyone watching, it looked as though we were old pals.

He did this for a few days. Then he charged in for the kill at an American Cancer Society luncheon in honor of Ted junior that, coincidentally, took place during the hearings. Kennedy and his wife were then in the papers every day because of their bitter divorce. I found myself seated at a long table, onstage, facing the audience, next to his soon to be ex-wife, Joan. At one point, Kennedy came over and pulled up a chair next to me and Joan. The cameras flashed so brightly, and so frequently, that I was blinded. I thought it was odd that he had a piece of paper in his right hand. He held it in front of me and looked at me while conversing with Joan. I didn't think all that much of it until the next day. The photograph—of Kennedy holding a piece of paper in front of me—was front-page news. The papers reported that I had given Kennedy a piece of paper on which was written confidential information related to the hearings. I hadn't, of course. But Kennedy had made me look suspicious.*

I was completely unprepared. My alleged leak angered Hatch so much that he called me in to see him and Frank Silbey, the chief investigator for the Senate Labor and Human Resources Committee. I assured Hatch that I hadn't leaked anything, but the photograph was pretty damning. After Hatch left, Silbey treated me to a withering speech. He told me he was going to leak false detrimental information about me to *The New York Times* and there wasn't a thing I could do about it. "As far as I'm concerned," he said, "you're dead meat."

Another staff member was within earshot during this diatribe, a passive, rotund guy named David Kessler, a future FDA commissioner

---

*After Senator Kennedy died, I was called by a reporter from *The Boston Globe* who said that he knew the senator had been a big supporter of the war on cancer and encouraged me to say something about that. I told the reporter that as far as I could remember, the senator had never done anything to support the war on cancer besides agreeing to step off the Senate bill as a sponsor to appease President Nixon. In fact, Senator Kennedy was instead a big supporter of the FDA and often its de facto one-man court of last resort. When I was negotiating with the FDA to develop the master plan for dealing with anticancer drugs, especially for making new drugs available for cancer patients before they were marketed, disgruntled FDA staffers regularly called the senator's office to complain. Senator Kennedy would then admonish me for attacking the FDA. When he was stricken with brain cancer, I was called, as were many of my colleagues, and asked by Kennedy staffers about gaining access to the newest agents for treating brain cancer. I told them I thought a vaccine developed at Duke Cancer Center was interesting. It was not available to the average patient, however. I do not know whether or not he gained access to it, but the medical community was quite surprised when he left one of the finest hospitals in Boston and had his care transferred to the Duke medical center.

and future dean of the School of Medicine at Yale. Apparently, Kessler felt sorry for me and convinced Hatch that I was innocent. Soon afterward, the hearings ended—with a thud, not a bang. I kept my job. And I was able to get back to work on cancer—which was, after all, what I was supposed to be doing.

In Greek mythology, there's a story referred to as "The Twelve Labors of Hercules" in which Hercules, driven mad by Hera, goes on a murderous rampage. When he comes to his senses, full of regret, he's told to perform twelve nearly impossible "labors" to atone for his sins. Looking at the list of things that needed to change at the NCI, I felt a vague sense of kinship with Hercules. One of his assigned labors was to clean out the Augean stable, home to a thousand immortal cattle, which had not been cleaned in more than thirty years. A thousand immortal cows produce a lot of dung.

I thought of that as I began my nearly impossible labor of reforming the way the NCI gave out research funds. This was going to be at least as tough a battle as those I'd already been through. Research supported by R01 grants was my number-one priority. Our future depended on it. R01 grants support young investigators starting a career in cancer research. They are the seed corn for future advances. When arguing for more support for research grants, I always remind people that everything we know that works came from research.

But this was not my only priority. In times of tight funding, it remained number one, but I adjusted the support to try to preserve the silhouette of the cancer program created by the cancer act and vital to its mandate to support research and the application of the results of research. I wasn't willing to strangle other vital parts of the NCI programs, such as cancer centers and clinical trials, for the sake of R01 grants. There was not much point in making advances if you didn't have the ability to apply them.

The NIH and the academic institutes didn't like it. They considered it a perversion of the scientific process. "Money can't buy ideas" was the common refrain. Universities didn't like it, either. Their entire academic promotion system was based on the attainment of R01 grants. Universities needed these grants to support their research faculty. So they would resist any change in the way the NIH did its business.

So there were plenty of critics, but the fact was that, in many instances, contracts worked. They were given with goals in mind and could be given faster than grants, which were awarded through a different peer review system. But contractors had the same freedom as grantees to pursue their day-to-day research projects within a general framework. No one from the NCI told them what to do each day.

The NCI had first used contracts very successfully with the drug-screening program that Zubrod had run to find drugs that might be effective against cancer. The Special Virus Cancer Program also relied on contracts. As I mentioned earlier, Congress had established the SVCP in 1964, at the urging of Mary Lasker, based on the fact that some scientists had reported finding virus-like particles in some cancer tissues with an electron microscope.

The mission of the Special Virus Cancer Program was to look for viruses that might cause cancer and then vaccinate people against them. By 1980, it was clear that those virus particles scientists had thought they saw were, in fact, false images produced by electron microscopy. Despite that, the program had churned out a startling array of findings. Viruses were, in fact, aiding us in the war on cancer. They'd helped us identify genes responsible for a cancer cell's ability to grow uncontrollably and commit suicide. The genes, and their products, gave us a new and highly specific range of targets for new cancer treatments. It was paradigm-changing work. The entire field of molecular biology owed its origins to such research, and six Nobel prizes would eventually be awarded to scientists who traced their original work back to the SVCP.

That was one reason the NCI liked contracts. Another was that the NCI's contracting authority was truly independent of the rest of the NIH.

But that wasn't to say that all contracts were good, and I suspected that some needed to be reviewed and possibly terminated. We were at war. We had to be serious, focused, disciplined, and most of all optimistic, and try to communicate the significance of the discoveries coming out of the NCI programs.

At that time, more than 20 percent of the NCI's billion-dollar budget was tied up in about twelve hundred research contracts. Sixty-five percent was tied up in R01 grants. The rest was in clinical research and the NCI's intramural programs. I wasn't happy about this, but that was what I'd inherited. I had to make the most of the 20 percent the NCI did have complete control over.

I'd made it clear that my first priority as director would be to examine each contract to determine if it was to stay, go, or be cut back. The review took about six weeks of nearly round-the-clock work. In the end, it was clear that some good work was being done with contracts, but a lot of money had gone to powerful figures who might—or might not—be doing the best research.

Some prominent intramural scientists at the NCI—that is, those who worked inside its walls—were using contracts as a source of money that would run not only their own labs but the labs of friends and associates. They set up what amounted to mini grant programs, providing largesse for colleagues outside the NCI. In fact, the SVCP, where so much landmark work had been done, was a prime offender.

This had started out as a defensive move. Because of the NIH's hostility toward research supported by contracts, the administrator who'd run it had clustered important scientists around the program—giving them lavish support in return for their collaboration.

The deal, I suspected, was that in return for the money, if an NCI director attempted to take the authority or funds away from the scientists who had the contract, the scientists on the dole would come out—seemingly just as good scientific citizens—and publicly attack the director by saying he just didn't understand or appreciate the science involved. Many on the dole were famous scientists whose critiques of others were especially effective precisely because of their prominence.

By the time I arrived on the scene, the SVCP had become almost like an institute within an institute, sucking up money that was needed for other new initiatives.

With the stroke of a pen, I converted the SVCP research contracts to grants. When the expiration date of the original contract came up, these investigators would have to submit a grant application to receive more funds. It didn't hurt the scientists who did well in the peer review system; it appealed to the sense of fairness of the other scientists who had been wary and envious of the use of sumptuous contracts for research; and it took away one of the major criticisms of the NCI—the use of contracts to accelerate research. It also left meritorious contracts we needed on the books and able to function without the daily criticism that was aimed at the source of their funding rather than the actual work being done.

I made equally dramatic changes elsewhere at the NCI—too many to describe here. But a few were particularly important.

In the history of cancer research, there has always been tension between those who want to treat cancer and those who think we should prevent it. Obviously, both are important. The question at the time was, where should researchers focus their efforts?

Activists who believed that chemicals in the environment were responsible for a large percentage of cancer regularly charged that there was a grand conspiracy to hide the evidence. Several epidemiologists had foisted a chemical-testing program on the NCI, overstating the impact of environmental chemicals as a cause of concern. The program was called the National Toxicology Program (NTP), and its mission was to search for cancer-causing chemicals by seeing whether suspected carcinogens would cause tumors in mice. Testing a single chemical took almost two years and thousands of mice. Because more than a million new chemical structures are estimated to be added to the world each year, testing any significant fraction of them for their cancer-causing properties in mice was not really possible. This led to some odd testing protocols, with mice being exposed to doses of chemicals hundreds or even a thousand times greater than any human would ever be exposed to.

This kind of testing often led to laughable results. The sweetener saccharin, for instance, was erroneously banned because it caused cancer in mice—at enormous doses. To get the same effect in humans, a person would have to drink several cases of a saccharin-containing soft drink a day for his entire life. This revelation led to cartoons of bloated mice lying next to cases and cases of diet soft drinks.

Also, mice are not like humans. There's no assurance that a chemical that's safe for mice is safe in humans—and vice versa. But somehow, the money funneled to this program kept expanding. By the time I became director, the budget for the NTP was $50 million. It employed eighty people and threatened to overwhelm research on more important causes of cancer, such as smoking and diet.

Clearly the people behind this program knew I had it in my sights, because among the first calls I got after my appointment was from one of the epidemiologists who'd spearheaded the NTP. He invited me to dinner at his favorite organic restaurant.

Dinner had scarcely begun when he started to threaten me. "I'm responsible for the budget of the NTP," he said, leaning over his plate. "Unless you play ball with me, I'll bleed the NCI to death. All your budget increases will go to us."

I decided to get rid of the program. The NIH had another institute, the National Institute of Environmental Health Sciences, located in Research Triangle Park, North Carolina, and it was directed by my former mentor Dave Rall. I thought the NTP belonged there, anyway. I met with Dave and Jim Wyngaarden, the NIH director, and told them my plans. They were shocked. No one in Washington ever gave away a program with that kind of money, let alone eighty treasured personnel slots. But I was serious, and the National Cancer

Advisory Board backed the transfer. Soon the NTP would no longer be my problem.

The second issue that occupied me around the same time was devising a better way to get research findings to doctors and patients. What good was the NCI's work if it wasn't making a difference to the cancer patients whose lives depended upon it?

Once again, Mary Lasker got involved.

When I was director of the Division of Cancer Treatment, Mary would come to my office with a computer printout a foot high from an NCI service called CLINPROT—government-speak for "clinical protocols." If you went to CLINPROT and pressed the print button, you had best get out of the way of your printer. Otherwise, you risked being swamped by paper. What you would get was a list of every NCI scientific study described in minute and indecipherable detail.

Mary didn't like it. "I asked for something useful for patients, and I got this instead," Mary said, disdainfully letting the accordion folds of the printout tumble to the floor. "Can't you do something?" she asked.

The printouts from CLINPROT would have challenged the patience of the most dedicated financial analysts and program directors at the NCI. We needed a computerized cancer information system to let doctors outside the institute know where studies were being done and what they were designed to find out. At the time, personal computers were just becoming widespread, and we had the computer power to make better use of all this information.

We began planning the new information resource in September 1982. We called it PDQ, for Physician Data Query. (It wasn't an accident that PDQ also stood for "pretty damned quick.")

I put a planning team together to design PDQ. We needed to assemble all the information on clinical trials into an easy-to-use database. We also decided to write up what we called state-of-the-art protocols describing each kind of cancer and how it should be treated. We asked for help from specialists inside and outside the NCI, and we got it. We set a target of less than two years for the completion of the project.

We quickly ran into a problem when we wanted to sign a contract that would send all of the work to a single contractor. By law, all contracts with the government need to be competed for in the open market. Giving contracts to your friends without competition was a source of corruption. To get a "sole source" contract approved was hell. You needed all kinds of departmental approvals, and even then it was frowned on. And the truth was, sometimes there was a case for them. In this case, in 1982, there truly was only one contractor with software that had touch screens and could do what we needed to do to set up PDQ. There was a provision in contract law that said you could go ahead with a contract without competition if the contractor was the "sole source" of that kind of work. We were planning on using it.

I called the PDQ team together to meet with a representative from the office of Margaret Heckler, the secretary of health and human services, who presided over both the NIH and the NCI. He was blunt and abrupt. He would not approve a sole-source contract. When I said I thought the NCI director had the authority to do it, he opened a manual with department regulations and pointed out that I could award the contract only if I was willing to declare a national emergency. He slammed the manual shut with a smug look on his face, satisfied that he had stopped us.

I stared at him for a minute, before doing the only thing I could. "I'm declaring a state of emergency," I said. "For every day we delay this system, someone is going to die unnecessarily." In my view, that more than justified the declaration. He was stunned and left without saying more. The next day, he came back with the necessary papers for me to sign. Weeks later, I went to a reception in Secretary Heckler's office for something else. Her chief of staff come over to me with a smile on his face. Our national emergency was the talk of the office, and they liked it, he said. He told me that the staffer who had confronted us had lost his son to leukemia. I wondered if

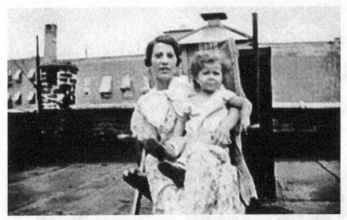

My favorite aunt, Violet, holding my older sister, Angela, in 1936. Aunt Violet died of cervical cancer at the age of thirty-six a few years after this picture was taken. Angela died of lung cancer in 2015, only months before the FDA approved a drug that might have helped her.

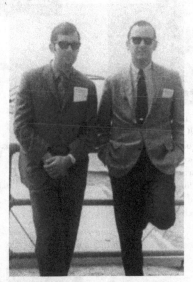

With Jack Moxley on the Atlantic City boardwalk, circa 1964. By this time, Moxley and I were midway through the MOMP trial that would lead to the first curative combination chemotherapy regimen for an adult cancer.

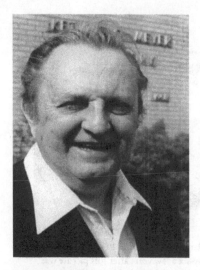

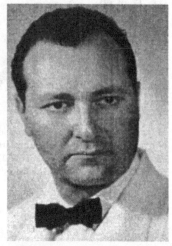

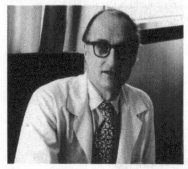

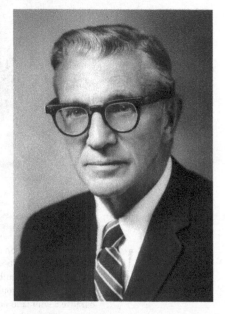

TOP Howard Skipper, the self-proclaimed mouse doctor of the NCI; ABOVE RIGHT Jay Freireich; ABOVE Tom Frei; RIGHT Gordon Zubrod (Credit: The Website of the National Cancer Institute, www.cancer.gov). Together, they revolutionized the treatment of childhood leukemia with combination chemotherapy.

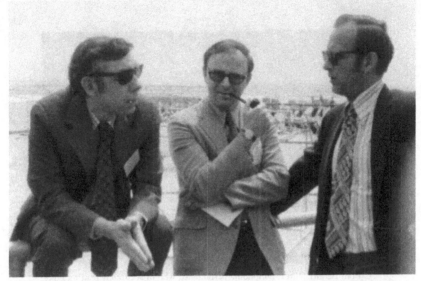

Back on the boardwalk with, from left to right, Ron Yankee, who helped me decipher the cell growth rates of leukemia in our mouse model, which would help me transform MOMP into MOPP; George Canellos, nicknamer extraordinaire; and Jack Moxley

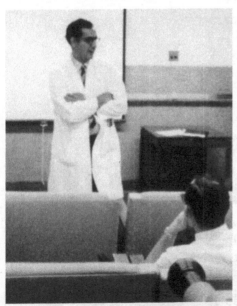

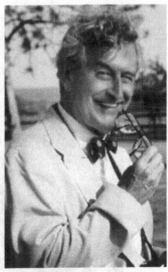

David Platt Rall, chief of chemical pharmacology at the NCI. He recruited me to the NCI while I was still a lowly medical student.

Paul Carbone, chief of the NCI's medicine branch at the time of this photo. The clinical associates gave him a terrible time—largely because he was easier to take on than the terrifying Jay Freireich. In truth, he was a good doctor and much beloved and admired by his peers.

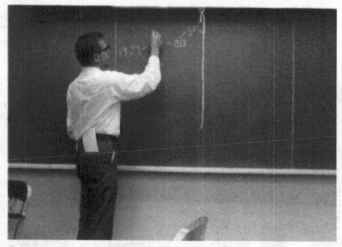

Costan Berard, a great lymphoma pathologist, who in accurately reading Luke Quinn's biopsy slides set a process in motion that would help trigger the war on cancer. Here he is at one of the blackboards in the room where the Society of Jabbering Idiots met to discuss our research.

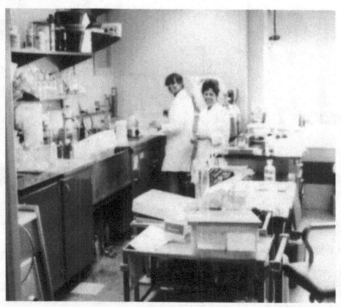

My lab, circa 1970. It was so small that I could reach most of what I needed without leaving my chair.

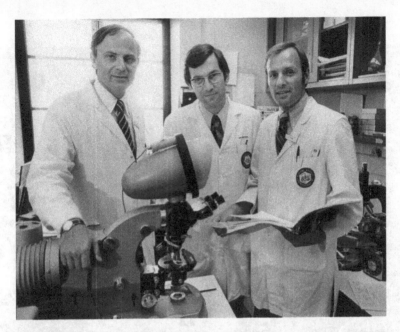

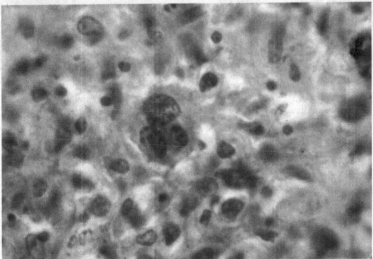

TOP George Canellos, Bob Young, and me, circa 1971. By this time, Canellos and I were working on combination chemotherapy for breast cancer, and I'd put Young in charge of the chemotherapy for early-stage Hodgkin's disease and the ovarian cancer program. (Credit: Joel Carl Freid)

ABOVE This is the cell that sparked my big breakthrough—the Reed-Sternberg cell, the one in the center with three nuclei. Seen through a microscope, it looks like an owl looking back at you. When this cell appears in a lymphoma, that's what makes it Hodgkin's disease—and it's what makes Hodgkin's a cancer. The slide pictured here is from one of the original six cases reported by Thomas Hodgkin in 1832.

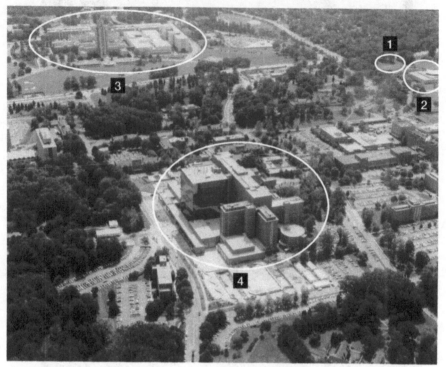

"The Chemo Trail."

1. The trail
2. National Library of Medicine
3. Bethesda Naval Hospital
4. NIH Building #10

The pioneering Hodgkin's patients who were the first to be treated with MOPP used to walk from the clinical center to their hotel because they knew that if they took the shuttle, they'd vomit. Thus they forged the Chemo Trail, which was later paved by the NIH.

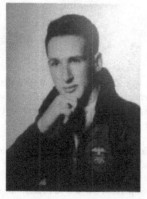

The man who told me about the Chemo Trail was Fred Feldman, one of the first patients on MOPP. He contracted Hodgkin's after he was overexposed to Agent Orange in Vietnam, around the time this picture was taken. He's still alive today. (Courtesy of Fred Feldman)

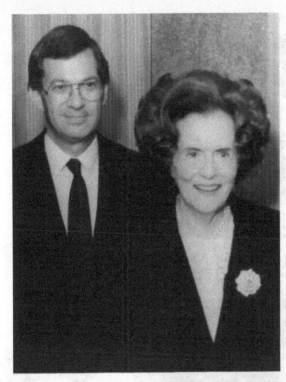

Mary Lasker decided we needed a war on cancer—and she made it happen. Her bouffant, mink coat, and ever-present compact could fool you into thinking she was just a socialite. Nothing could have been further from the truth.

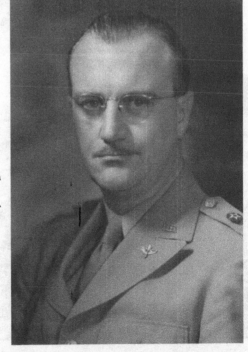

Colonel Luke C. Quinn in the late 1940s. His case tipped Mary Lasker into a full-blown effort to launch the war on cancer. (Courtesy of Colonel Luke C. Quinn's family)

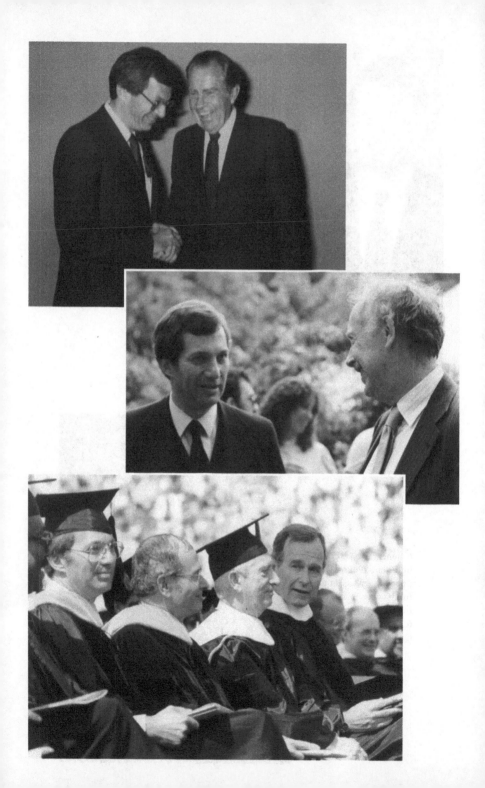

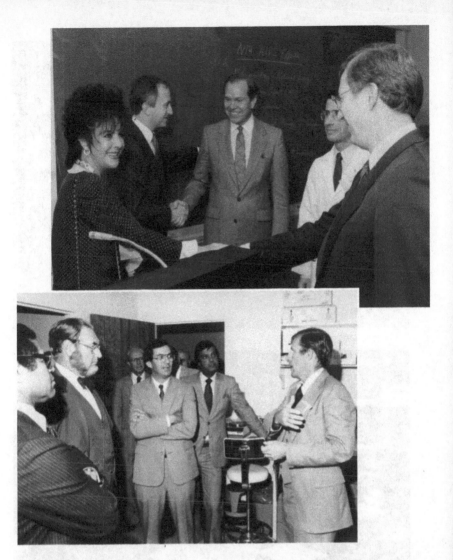

After the National Cancer Act was passed, the relatively quiet area of cancer research became political. Sometimes members of the NCI were summoned to make appearances in Washington. At other times, political figures came to see us. TOP LEFT With former president Richard Nixon. I asked him what he thought were the greatest achievements of his presidency. He said going to China and signing the National Cancer Act. MIDDLE LEFT With the Nobel Prize winner Jim Watson, a brilliant scientist with apparently little understanding of the role and value of clinical research (that doesn't stop him from making erroneous predictions about cures to the press, however) (Credit: Joan James). BOTTOM LEFT With former president George H. W. Bush, who has a long-standing interest in cancer research—he lost a young daughter to leukemia (Official White House Photograph). TOP Elizabeth Taylor, who had an interest in the NIH's AIDS program, then located at both NCI and NIAID, shaking hands with me, while Terry Lierman shakes hands with the NIH's director, James Wyngaarden, third from the left, and the NIAID director, Anthony Fauci, in white lab coat, looks on. ABOVE Former surgeon general C. Everett Koop taking a tour.

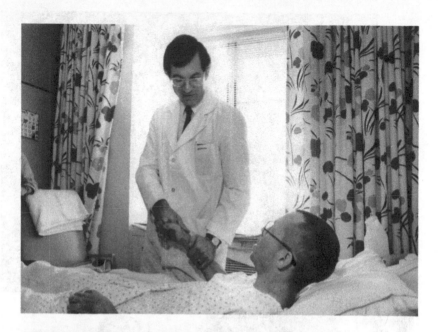

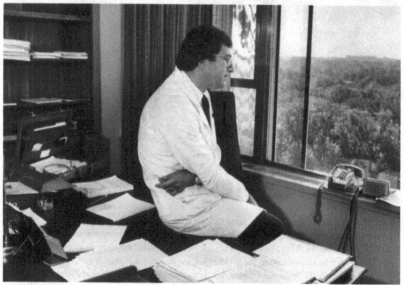

TOP With a patient on 12 West. I loved taking care of patients, and this was one of the hardest things for me to give up when I became the director of the NCI. Whenever the politics and the administrative work of the war on cancer became overwhelming, I'd take time to make rounds to visit with the patients. It always clarified my priorities—and made me feel better. (Credit: Diana Walker for *People*)

ABOVE Looking out the window of my office, after I had become director of the NCI. The job was vital to the success of the war on cancer, but it could be a crusher. (Credit: Diana Walker for *People*)

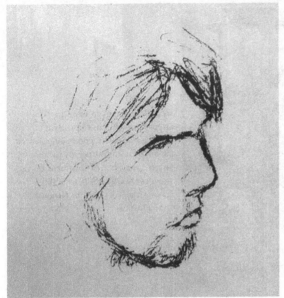

A self-portrait done by my son, Ted, who died at seventeen after a nearly eight-year battle with aplastic anemia. Ted's diagnosis, illness, and death taught me what it really means to wait for a cure that is too slow to arrive.

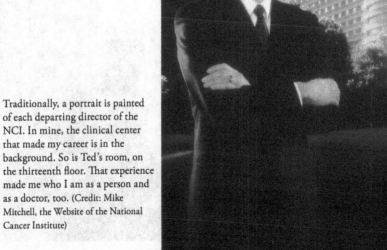

Traditionally, a portrait is painted of each departing director of the NCI. In mine, the clinical center that made my career is in the background. So is Ted's room, on the thirteenth floor. That experience made me who I am as a person and as a doctor, too. (Credit: Mike Mitchell, the Website of the National Cancer Institute)

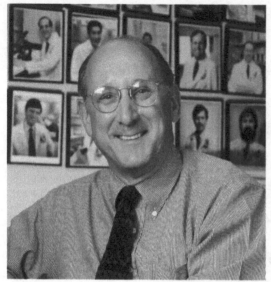

Steve Rosenberg, chief of the NCI's surgery branch. He's a brilliant physician-scientist who revolutionized the use of immunotherapy in treating cancer, an avenue of treatment that's only now taking off. (Credit: Bill Branson, the Website of the National Cancer Institute)

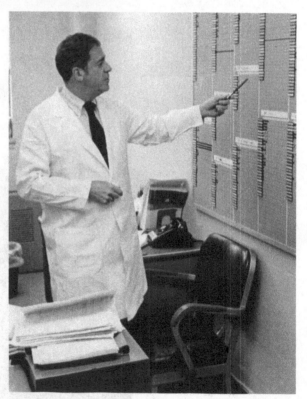

The great Bernie Fisher, circa 1960. Bernie faced the wrath of his fellow surgeons when he proved that lumpectomy was as effective as mastectomy in treating breast cancer. He's one of those rare doctors who's willing to challenge the status quo to do what's right on behalf of patients.

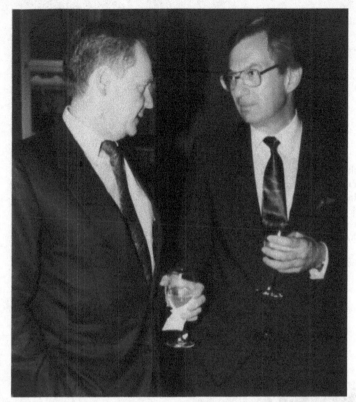

Having a drink with Murray Brennan, then chief of surgery at Memorial Sloan Kettering Cancer Center. Murray is possibly the most skilled surgeon I've ever met. I would scrub in on operations just to watch him work.

Zvi Fuks, chief of radiotherapy at MSKCC when I was there, and one of the most skilled and adventurous radiotherapists I've ever known

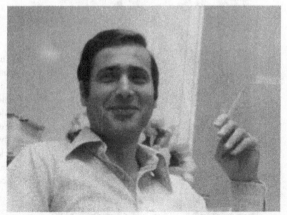

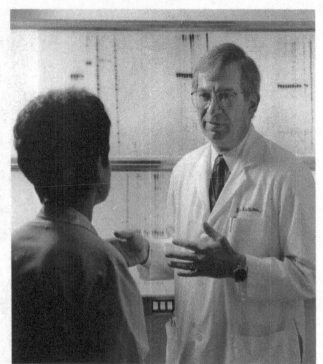

Talking over lab results with a researcher at Yale. On the viewbox behind me are her electrophoretic gels, which separate molecules by size and electric charge. (© Robert A. Lisak)

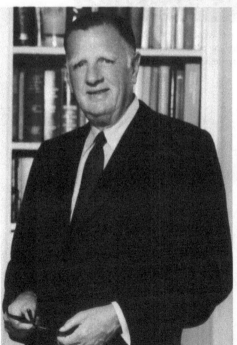

Benno C. Schmidt, who was a managing partner at J. H. Whitney and the chair of the President's Cancer Panel, which would help plot the course for the war on cancer. Schmidt could analyze some scientific issues more quickly than many scientists. (Credit: The Website of the National Cancer Institute)

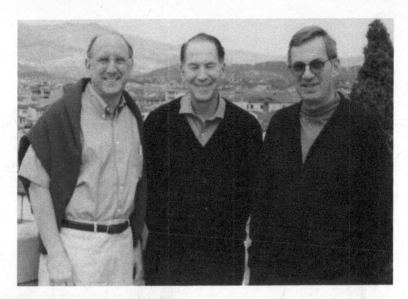

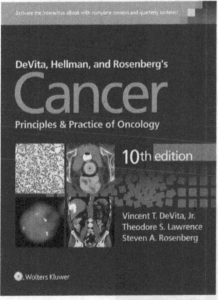

ABOVE Steve Rosenberg, Sam Hellman, and me while we were editing our textbook, *Cancer: Principles & Practice of Oncology*. All three of us had strong opinions and we were not shy about expressing them, but we became so comfortable working together that doing the book was a joy. Our debates made it the most comprehensive and reliable text on the subject in the world.

LEFT The most recent edition of our textbook, the only online continuously updated oncology textbook in existence (DeVita, Lawrence, and Rosenberg, *Cancer: Principles & Practices of Oncology*, 10th edition, Wolters Kluwer, 2014)

BELOW Jay Freireich and me reminiscing about old times at a recent meeting of the American Society of Clinical Oncology. What he taught me in the 1960s still holds true for both of us: you never give up on a patient.

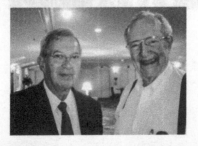

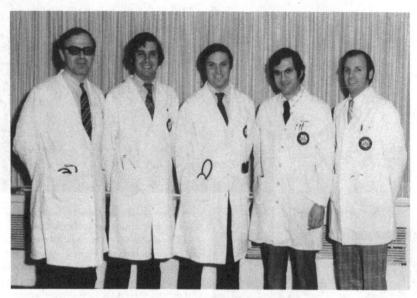

The gang of five at the medicine branch in 1973 (*above*) and forty years later in 2013 (*below*). From left to right: George Canellos, Bruce Chabner, Philip Schein, me, and Robert Young

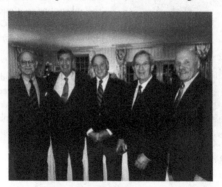

his son had missed out on one of the new therapies for childhood leukemia; I never learned the full story. We issued the contract and got immediate access to both the software and the hardware we needed.

The job of the NCI director, when done right, was a crusher. From time to time, I found myself feeling mildly depressed. When that happened, my therapy was to put time aside to make regular rounds on the cancer floors. After a month of this, my spirits would lift again. Some of my friends thought I was nuts. "How can making rounds on a ward full of cancer patients make you less depressed?" they asked. "Shouldn't it be the reverse?" Not for me. It reminded me why I was doing what I was doing. Rebuilding the NCI wasn't a bureaucratic exercise; it was about saving lives.

One day in 1984, I got a call from a distressed Bernie Fisher, the pioneering breast cancer researcher at the University of Pittsburgh. He led a team that had done a remarkable study comparing outcomes after mastectomy and lumpectomy and found no difference between the two. But he couldn't get the study published. It had been tied up in review at *The New England Journal of Medicine* for almost nine months, and the reviewers still weren't finished evaluating it.

Every paper submitted to the top medical journals gets reviewed by peers, who judge its scientific merits and decide whether it should be published. The process can take months, but nine months was unusually long—especially for a study that would have an immediate impact on the way breast cancer was treated. This would be a profound change. The longer the study was held up, the more women would have unnecessarily aggressive surgery for breast cancer.

Bernie's study was controversial, because breast surgeons made their living doing radical or total mastectomies, and they did not want to hear that that was no longer necessary. Fisher had found it difficult to get patients referred to his study, in fact, because of this resistance. Doctors refused to participate. Bernie and I had actually made the rounds on morning TV shows to present the findings to the public.

After every show, a few more patients were referred. Now the study results, which changed the paradigm for breast cancer treatment, were being delayed, possibly for the same old reason—resentment. Bernie suspected his study was being deliberately held up by reviewers who themselves resented the change in practice that it was suggesting.

Fisher didn't know where to turn. "Is there anything you can do?" he asked me.

I knew Bud Relman, the editor of *The New England Journal of Medicine*, and I gave him a call. I asked why the paper was being held so long. Was Bernie right about surgeons' resentment and unwillingness to accept the findings? "Vince, that's impossible," Bud told me. "But let me check. Hold on."

Five minutes later, Bud was back. "My God, it's true," he said. The study had been sent out to surgical colleagues for review—five of them, which was three more than usual. It was first sent to two, who didn't think it should be published. Their biggest claim was that not enough time had passed to draw any conclusions, and the radical mastectomy, by contrast, had seventy-five years of follow-up. The reviewers had also accused Fisher of being unethical and argued that all patients should get a radical until we knew otherwise. They also claimed that it must be that ordinary surgeons doing radical mastectomies probably weren't doing a good job, which accounted for why the radical was not faring better compared with the less radical surgery.

I'd heard these arguments before, and they were easy to demolish if you paid attention.

But the surgeons who'd received the paper for review were big names, so *The New England Journal of Medicine* just kept sending it out to more breast surgeons with the same result. Such was the influence of powerful surgeons. Not because the science was bad, but because they didn't want to give up the more extensive surgery that created 90 percent of their income. It was economics. I got the same kind of response when I suggested in a talk that we needed to stop routine postoperative radiotherapy for breast cancer. A radiotherapist came up to me and said, "What am I supposed to do? One-third of my practice is postoperative radiotherapy for breast cancer. If we stop doing it, I'd have to lay off one of our radiotherapists." Most surgeons and radiotherapists would never admit that they opposed Fisher's findings because they threatened the doctors' incomes. Instead, they questioned his integrity. That's why Relman and his editors had sent it out to three more reviewers.

I explained to Bud that I thought the problem was resistance from surgeons. And I reminded him how many thousands of women in the United States and around the world were being deprived of the option to have less extensive surgery—all because the paper languished at the journal. The paper was published six weeks later.

I wondered how often this kind of thing happened. If the illustrious Bernie Fisher had problems getting published, what happened to people who didn't have an intermediary they could call upon to intervene, as I had done for Bernie? That's when I got the idea to issue the NCI clinical alerts. I decided that we would take it upon ourselves to release data from game-changing papers as soon as they were reviewed and accepted by a journal but before publication.

Three years later, in 1987, I got the first opportunity to try this with another study by Bernie and his team that was wending its way slowly through the review process. The study looked at the use of postoperative chemotherapy in breast cancer patients in whom cancer cells had not spread to the lymph nodes. The study had found that in patients with tumors greater than two centimeters in diameter, chemotherapy prolonged survival, even if it appeared that the cancer had not spread to the lymph nodes. In other words, patients who might otherwise have been given the all clear and sent home without additional therapy after surgery did better if you added chemotherapy to their treatment plan. Like Fisher's earlier study, this one was paradigm changing. I thought other doctors and the public needed to know about it as soon as possible. About five thousand women in the United States who fell in this category had surgery each year, and many would miss the benefits of post-op chemotherapy if we waited for publication.

I called Bernie and told him about my clinical alert idea and said I wanted to use it for his study. He was reluctant, for fear it would jeopardize the paper's publication. *The New England Journal of Medicine* had a strict policy that it would not publish anything that had appeared elsewhere first—including in the popular press. I called Bud Relman again and asked if issuing a prepublication alert would make him withdraw the paper. "Not if the NCI thinks it's a matter of public health," he said.

We issued the first clinical alert in May 1987, two weeks before the annual meeting of the American Society of Clinical Oncology, otherwise known as ASCO. It went to thousands of physicians, many of whom were going to the ASCO meeting. We issued a press release shortly after the alert so that if curious patients asked their doctors about the treatment, doctors wouldn't be caught without the information.

I had no doubt that it was the right thing to do, but many oncologists didn't agree. Several doctors spotted me on the plane en route to Atlanta for ASCO and took the opportunity to tell me how wrong I was not to wait for publication so the peer review process could be completed. That is, so readers and the journal could be sure the study was legitimate and that the data supported the conclusions. Others raised questions at the ASCO business meeting, where I was asked to explain myself. I pointed out that by the time such articles were published, the data had been reviewed by hundreds of people at the NCI and other institutions, where the studies took place. I thought saving lives was more important. And patients, after all, had paid for these studies with their tax dollars and deserved an early look at the data. Putting the patient first was what the mandate of the cancer act was all about.

I didn't change the critics' minds, but I didn't care. I didn't need their permission to send out clinical alerts, and I intended to continue. Years later, the Rand Corporation did a study on the use of chemotherapy in women after surgery, and it noted not only that post-op chemotherapy was being used widely but that there had been a noticeable drop in mortality from breast cancer in this group. Rand attributed that to the NCI clinical alert.[2]

By the mid-1980s, I had completely reorganized the NCI and

made it over in the image proposed in the National Cancer Act. While criticism of the war on cancer continued, it was no longer aimed at the management of the NCI. A significant number of people—including the NCI's own biostatisticians, led by Dr. Marvin Schneiderman— projected that mortality rates from cancer would increase in linear fashion all the way out beyond the year 2000. Schneiderman and I had been at loggerheads over statistics for years. He loved to make straight-line projections of mortality from all cancers combined, which when projected to the year 2000 was a straight line going up, up, and away.

When I became the DCT director, I objected, because such projections obscured any progress we were making with less common cancers. Schneiderman and I got into big arguments about it. His philosophy was that if you go to Congress with bad news, you get more money than if you go showing progress. I thought the reverse and said so in public. But Rauscher and then Upton wouldn't ask him to change. When I became the NCI director, one of the first things I did was to reverse this policy and have the NCI report mortality rates by disease and by age groups. (By 1990, mortality rates had begun to drop and have continued to drop since then.)

I saw things differently. I knew we were seeing significant declines in mortality rates in cancers for which we had developed effective tools for diagnosis and treatment. We could anticipate some impact on cancer incidence with dietary modification programs and those that helped smokers to quit. And, of course, we were discovering new chemotherapy drugs and protocols all the time.

But we still had a problem: treatment was lagging behind the research. Many people who could benefit from the new research were not getting those benefits. There was a huge gap between what might be achieved in an ideal world and what was actually happening. Many women, for example, were still not getting adjuvant treatment for breast cancer. So we at the NCI decided to establish goals that would hopefully spur wide knowledge of and use of new therapies. We drafted goals for the year 2000 in cancer prevention, diagnosis, and treatment. We were startled to see that with a wide application of *what we already knew worked,** it would be theoretically possible to reduce cancer mortality rates by as much as 50 percent by that time.

A simple example of what we could do in goal setting is the use of breast cancer screening. In 1984, we were only screening 14 percent of eligible women with mammography. Our experts said that with a full-court press we might be able to achieve a top screening rate of around 70 percent, and that would have a predictable impact on breast cancer mortality. Given the time lapse between screening and impact on mortality rates, we would need to get to that level of screening by 1992, which we did, and screening has led to a significant decline in breast cancer mortality. I took a lot of heat for that prediction. I felt what we had done had a solid scientific basis, but it was unusual for a

---

*Screening for any cancer has often promised more than it can deliver. But for many years, that's all we had. It's also always difficult to argue that finding a cancer early is not beneficial. In truth, we have very few data from carefully controlled trials that show screening reduces mortality. It's not there, for example, in prostate cancer, barely detectable in cervical cancer because of a decrease in incidence, and controversial for breast cancer below the age of fifty.

In breast cancers, some small tumors are so aggressive that picking them up while small makes no difference in survival. No matter how often you screen, it would make no difference. And some tumors detected early are so benign they would never cause the patient's death, but the patient carries the burden of the diagnosis for life. It's also assumed that there is no risk to screening, but there is, including death from unnecessary procedures.

Also, the management of breast cancer is changing rapidly. People who tout screening like to create the impression that all the decline in mortality from breast cancer is due to early detection, but this is not so. Two-thirds of the reduction in mortality from breast cancer is due to the effectiveness of adjuvant drug treatment after surgery or radiotherapy. As treatment continues to improve, the relevance of screening diminishes, and recommendations should change.

The recent recommendations of the U.S. Preventive Services Task Force (USPSTF) to back off on the frequency of mammographies to every two years beginning at age fifty and ending at age seventy-four reflects the changing landscape. They differ from the ACS recommendations for annual screening starting at age forty, but as this book goes to print, the ACS is assembling a group to reexamine its own recommendations. My guess is they will come out in the direction of those made by the USPSTF.

None of these recommendations prevent patients from being screened by mammography at any age, at any frequency, if the patient and her doctor, after discussions of the pros and cons, feel it is necessary. And, of course, they don't apply for patients at increased risk of developing breast cancer.

government agency to make such a specific, testable prediction. Yet somebody needed to take the risk.

The NCI of course had no control over which cancer treatments were actually employed except through the use of the bully pulpit. We made a cautious prediction that a more realistic assessment would be a decline in mortality rates in the range of 15 to 25 percent for all cancers. We published these deliberations in an NCI monograph titled *Cancer Control Objectives for the Nation: 1985–2000*, and again the reaction was one of disbelief.[3]

Even something as simple as providing dietary advice proved to be a challenge. One of the things we thought was important to prevent colon cancer was getting enough fiber in the diet. To spread the word, we persuaded the Kellogg Company to put an announcement of our new plans for diet and prevention on the backs of packages of Kellogg's All-Bran cereal and in its TV ads. We did our own advertising blitz in cooperation with Kellogg, thus taking advantage of some $40 million in advertising we could not fund ourselves.

I was pleased with the success of this program until I got an urgent call from Jim Wyngaarden, the director of the NIH. He told me to come to his office immediately. I ran over to his building and found four staffers from the FDA, including the deputy commissioner, sitting grimly in a circle. They had told Jim that the NCI (and I, specifically) had violated their regulations by promoting a cereal to prevent cancer. They were anticipating going into supermarkets and removing all boxes of Kellogg's All-Bran from the shelves. In addition, the deputy commissioner patted his breast coat pocket and said he had a regulatory letter for me, because I had initiated this project.

This was serious business. A regulatory letter would ban me from any FDA-sponsored work and require me to resign as the NCI director. Wyngaarden had an amused look on his face, reminiscent of Jay Freireich's when he was watching a tug-of-war unfold. He told the FDA staffers that we hadn't promoted any product; we had merely used products to spread our message, and it would look pretty silly if FDA SWAT teams were photographed attacking All-Bran in supermarkets.

It wouldn't help when it became clear the agency was punishing the NCI director for trying to promote cancer prevention. They left, looking crestfallen. The deputy commissioner still had the regulatory letter in his breast pocket. Luckily, nothing ever came of it.

In August 1988, Paul Marks, the president of Memorial Sloan Kettering Cancer Center, phoned to see if I was interested in coming to New York to be the physician in chief of Memorial Hospital. The call caught me by surprise. I had gone to the NCI intending to stay for two years and had worked there for twenty-six. I'd been the longest-serving director in the history of the institute. I'd fought more battles than I'd ever dreamed were possible. I had been spending three months each year for the past fifteen years preparing and testifying before Congress. I'd become adept at it all, but I'd become weary of it, too.

I was also increasingly disappointed with government. Congress and the presidents under whom I'd served had little interest in the war on cancer. I understood Mary's reasoning in getting the government involved, and I did not think she was wrong. But I was tired of the politics that had come to surround cancer once the politicians had become part of the process. And Mary, the war on cancer's biggest defender, was not what she once was. She had had a stroke in 1981, and while she had recovered, she had never been quite the same. There was no one who could take her place. In November, we would have another presidential election, and if a Democrat won, I'd probably be booted out anyway. Nixon's war on cancer, now approaching the twenty-year mark, had launched an entirely new level of research on both normal and cancerous cells. New discoveries occurred in two alternating waves: first the development of new technology, then the use of that new technology to unravel the mysteries of developmental biology—the cells' inner lives. The techniques of molecular biology allowed us to break up DNA and search for individual genes—including those that cause cancer. We had used the wealth of research funds and had pried open the black box that was the cancer cell. Now we could peer in and watch the gears go around.

I'd done my best in my role as leader of the war on cancer. I'd jettisoned the palace guard and appointed new branch chiefs and division directors. I'd put research support on a secure footing, remodeled the NCI's clinical trials program, given cancer centers new direction, and taken steps to spread the results of our research to doctors and the public. I'd made all the tough decisions. The war on cancer was operating the way the National Cancer Act had said it should. I was done.

I thought about this while deciding what to tell Paul Marks at Sloan Kettering. I'd never been all that interested in money, but I was now fifty-three years old, and government salaries were low. I had begun to think about making a change so I could earn enough to secure my retirement.

I had been offered other jobs over the years, but they hadn't been interesting enough, for one reason or another. Sloan Kettering was different. It was a big cancer center—one of the prototypes for the other cancer centers in the country and probably the most famous cancer hospital in the world. I liked the challenge of focusing my energies on a single institution rather than on the whole world. And the salary Marks offered was four times what I was making at the NCI.

I announced my resignation to President Reagan and other officials connected with the NCI on August 15, 1988.

Much to my surprise, the director of the NIH, when announcing my retirement, said, "Vince DeVita is the best institute director NIH has ever had." Considering how often we had clashed, I thought that was a great compliment.

By September 1, I was retired from the U.S. Public Health Service at the rank of rear admiral. Although my wife, Mary Kay, is a painter, I decided I'd go for a photograph to commemorate my time in office, unlike Upton. In the image, I'm standing with my arms crossed, and the NIH Clinical Center, which made my career, is the backdrop. Only those closest to me know the additional meaning of the picture. What had once been our son's window is visible, in the background, over my left shoulder.

8

FRANCES KELSEY SYNDROME

When I left the NCI, I was proud of what I had done to reshape it into an organization capable of managing the war on cancer. But one challenge had eluded me: I was unable to persuade the administrators at the Food and Drug Administration to change the way they reviewed new cancer drugs. What might work when it came to a new diabetes drug or a cholesterol-lowering pill did not work for cancer drugs. The FDA's failure to recognize this was impeding our progress. And patients who could have been saved were dying.

Admittedly, the FDA has the most difficult job of all government agencies. Whatever it does, it receives a barrage of criticism. The world outside the FDA seems to be split into two groups. The first includes the many lawyers, doctors, and activists who want every aspect of our food and our drugs to be examined in fine detail before being approved so that we can eliminate as many potential risks as possible. The second group again includes lawyers, doctors, and activists, but this group holds that new drugs are too tightly regulated and that we should relax regulations so we can get potentially lifesaving drugs to patients sooner. Many members of this second group also believe that what we eat is none of the FDA's business.

If the FDA approves drugs rapidly, it angers the first group. If the FDA approves them too slowly, it angers the second. Of course, both groups have taken things too far. Most of us recognize that we need regulations; we don't want the FDA to go away. But we do want it to get out of the way. We need some regulations, but we don't need all that we have now.

Here's an example of what I mean: aspirin, one of our truly miracle drugs. In its early testing, it produced adenomas (small benign tumors) in the lungs of mice. Nothing like that has been seen in humans, but if aspirin were being developed today, the presence of adenomas might prevent the pill's approval. Aspirin, like all drugs, has some risks, but that doesn't mean we should take it out of patients' hands.

The FDA has brought criticism on itself by seeking (and getting) more and more control over our lives. Twenty-five percent of every dollar we spend in the United States goes to a product regulated by the FDA. The agency has more authority and control over our lives than almost any other government agency. Yet it still wants more.

When it comes to cancer, the FDA has reached far beyond its central responsibility—assuring the safety of new drugs. It is now regulating research and the practice of oncology—something it was never meant to do and is not capable of doing. In this chapter, I want to tell you how this happened and what I've tried to do about it.

In 2000, soon after President George W. Bush was elected, Donald Evans, his new commerce secretary, asked if I was interested in becoming the FDA commissioner. He was leading the president's search for a new commissioner. I hesitated; I knew how important it would be to have an FDA commissioner who had an open mind and experience with drug development. But I said no. This caught Secretary Evans by surprise. He expected me to at least say that I wanted to think about it. But I had thought about it. I had watched FDA commissioners come and go, and none seemed to have much impact on the way the FDA operated.

An FDA commissioner, above all, needs the courage of his or her convictions. If you can't please everybody, you should at least try to do what you believe to be the right thing. But most FDA commissioners try to please everybody. They become overly cautious and too vulnerable to entrenched interests at the middle level of the FDA. These bureaucrats are capable of scuttling the careers of commissioners—and do.

The mid-level FDA staffers are all of one mindset: they are for more regulations. In general, they think the FDA should move slowly and be extremely careful with new drugs. If they see that a commissioner is not sympathetic to this regulatory mission, they surreptitiously run to Congress to make their case.

Until recently, the late senator Ted Kennedy was their champion. When I was at the NCI, I would occasionally be called to Kennedy's office—usually when the NCI was having a dustup with the FDA. Phone calls from Larry Horowitz, his longtime staffer, or meetings with Kennedy himself were ways of warning me away every time I publicly went after the FDA for slowing down cancer drug development. If the weather was nice, we would sit on the balcony outside Kennedy's Senate office. I would stare at my own image reflected in his sunglasses, and he would tell me that going after the FDA was displeasing to him. I would try to explain where I was coming from, but he wasn't interested in hearing what I had to say. I just kept on doing what I thought was best for the cancer patients and the NCI.

The FDA commissioner has another challenge. As a presidential appointee, the commissioner not only has to contend with the pressure applied by mid-level FDA staff but also faces potential pressure from the White House to approve or disapprove drugs that have political implications—especially those related to birth control. I didn't need that headache, either.

During my time at the NCI, I worked with five different FDA

commissioners. The first four lasted only two years each. None was very helpful to the NCI, and none had much impact on how the FDA functioned.

Laws controlling the quality of imported foods and medicines have been in place in the United States since 1848. The first set of laws specifically related to drugs was passed in 1906, but it was not until 1927, when the Food, Drug, and Insecticide Administration was formed, that a specific government entity was charged with reviewing and approving drugs. Since then, the agency, largely in response to crises that alarmed the public (and, as a consequence, Congress), has assumed the most sweeping powers of any U.S. government agency.

The first memorable crisis occurred in 1937, when 107 people were killed from exposure to a chemical relative of antifreeze, diethylene glycol, that was used as a solvent in an elixir of the antibiotic sulfanil-amide. In response, Congress passed the U.S. Food, Drug, and Cosmetic Act in 1938, which required the manufacturers of drugs, for the first time, to prove their products were safe for human use. That was a good and necessary regulatory power.

The 1938 act also expanded the power of the FDA over cosmetics and medical devices, neither of which had anything to do with the sulfanilamide scandal. This was an FDA power grab, the first of many.

When Congress passes a law, the agency responsible for implementing it must write regulations detailing exactly how it will meet the law's requirements. These regulations are published in the *Federal Register*, and the agency can then get to work. The problem is that these regulations are often stiffer than the law itself. This is what happened with the FDA after the 1938 act. Over the next several years, the FDA extended its authority far beyond the original intent of Congress. It established drug-classification regulations that said, among other things, that some drugs could be dispensed by prescription only. It asked for and received authority over interstate commerce in drugs, cosmetics, and devices. And it required that manufacturers, in their applications for drug approvals, state the purpose for which a drug would be used.

This was the basis for the FDA's control over unapproved, or off-label, uses for approved drugs. Under the current regulations, the FDA can approve a drug for, say, one kind of cancer but restrict the use of the drug for another kind of cancer. This has proved highly detrimental to the post-marketing development of anticancer drugs. Why? Because we always learn more about how to use new cancer drugs in research studies done *after* the drugs are approved. In this so-called post-marketing period, investigators often uncover additional activity against cancer. The treatments that cured leukemia, Hodgkin's disease, and breast cancer were developed in just this manner. Innovative and experienced clinical researchers who want to propose new studies are at the mercy of FDA staffers—many of whom are not trained as cancer doctors, let alone as clinical researchers.

So far-reaching, and so controversial, were these new FDA regulations that the agency feared legal challenges could undo them. So it pushed Congress to write the regulation into the law, and in 1951 Congress amended the 1938 act to do exactly that.

The FDA continued its reach into the lives of Americans. In 1959, when the U.S. cranberry crop was recalled three weeks before Thanksgiving because of contamination with the chemical aminotriazole, a weed killer, the FDA exercised the power of seizure. It became a full-fledged law enforcement agency. In fact, the FDA commissioner carries a badge just like a cop. This point was brought home to me on many occasions in later years when the FDA commissioner Frank Young, annoyed by my public criticism of his agency at National Cancer Advisory Board meetings, used to flash his badge and remind me that he had arresting powers. He was speaking only half in jest.

While I am no friend of the FDA, I understand the agency's history, which helps to explain why it has been so eager to regulate research and practice and has been hypercautious in providing access to new drugs. Oddly, the roots of this caution can be found in what is usually regarded as a huge FDA success.

The story begins in 1960, when the FDA received an application for a drug called thalidomide for treating morning sickness. Frances Kelsey, a new drug reviewer at the agency, got the assignment. Kelsey was a Canadian-born physician and Ph.D. pharmacologist who, before she was hired by the FDA, had helped the FDA show that the diethylene glycol solvent used for sulfanilamide, taken for common infections, was responsible for 107 deaths, leading the agency to ban it.[1]

Kelsey took a careful look at thalidomide. It had already been approved in Canada and some twenty other European and African countries as an antiemetic and soporific (it both suppressed nausea and induced sleep) under the trade name Kevadon. Another reviewer might have approved the drug, on the assumption that it had undergone sufficient evaluation and needed only cursory review in the United States, but Kelsey, upon discovering an English study that found some effects on the nervous system, insisted on further studies. While the drug's approval was being delayed so those studies could be done, infants with severe limb abnormalities were born in Europe, and the problems were quickly linked to thalidomide. In a 1962 front-page story in *The Washington Post*, Kelsey was called a hero for averting similar tragic incidents in the United States. President Kennedy gave her a medal.[2]

It was, indeed, a good call. Pregnant women should avoid taking any drugs they absolutely don't need, especially new drugs with unknown side effects, because the rapidly growing body of a fetus is so susceptible to damage. And preclinical testing is not routinely done in pregnant animals to determine if a drug causes birth defects. Nor (thankfully) do most drug trials include pregnant women. If there ever was a case of being in the right place at the right time, this was it.

Up to that point, the FDA had based its approvals on whether a drug was held to be safe. Now Congress added a new criterion: in order to gain approval, drugs had to be shown not only to be safe but to be effective. Determination of effectiveness was not the issue in the thalidomide near-debacle. The issue there was safety. But once more, the FDA managed to make a power grab.

Thalidomide had actually been shown to be effective at treating morning sickness—which is why it had been approved in twenty countries. It had passed review because the defect noted by Kelsey, who was trained to look for these defects, had been missed by reviewers in other countries. While she deserved the acclaim that she received, it should not have been used to support what I have called "Frances Kelsey syndrome."

The thalidomide episode sent the message to those who worked at the FDA that the way to do right by people was to say no. Saying yes could prove perilous—not only to patients, but to the career of a re-viewer. As a result, the agency tends to reward those who say no, not yes. (In fact, there's an annual Frances Kelsey award. But there are no awards for getting a good drug quickly into the public domain.)

A legion of "Dr. No's" has been created, and they're particularly prone to saying no to cancer drugs. That's very bad news for cancer patients. Also bad news: Under the Kefauver-Harris Amendment, or "Drug Efficacy Amendment," of 1962, proof of efficacy was to be de-termined in "adequate and well controlled trials." The act mentions only the use of historical controls—that is, data from previous studies. The amendment did not require new randomized controlled trials, as people often think. The requirement for these new trials—often an unnecessary impediment in early drug trials—was added by the FDA in its interpretation of the regulations: another FDA grab.

Today we seem to be mindlessly wedded to the use of random-ized controlled trials. They have their place. But randomized clinical trials can be unethical. Doctors sometimes have strong beliefs about the effectiveness of treatments being compared in a randomized trial—often with good reason. And if they truly believe that the treatments are effective—while a placebo given to some patients is not—then it is their duty as physicians to tell patients so. Not many physicians take this position, but they should.

As it happens, we recently had a good example of this. In 2008, a new drug then known as PLX4032 was under study for metastatic melanoma—the malignant mole. Melanoma, when widespread, was almost invariably fatal, and there had been no drug that really worked in this condition, although the standard treatment is a drug called dacarbazine, approved years ago by the FDA. Frankly, everyone who has cared for patients with melanoma and treated them with dacarbazine knows it really doesn't work.

PLX4032, on the other hand, was producing startling results. Part of a new wave of targeted treatments now being developed, PLX4032 was a drug that, for the first time in my memory, produced good-quality responses in most patients who got it. The majority of patients responded to it, and a substantial number went into complete remission. And it was safe—much safer than dacarbazine. No one had seen a drug do this before in melanoma. It was prolonging survival and providing a better quality of life with few of dacarbazine's side effects. You might ask why dacarbazine was approved in the first place. At the time, it showed promise, but not much. Yet because there was nothing else, it was approved. But unless someone figures out a new way to use it that makes it effective, it has had enough years of testing to indicate that, by itself, it is nearly worthless.

Despite the promising results with PLX4032, in 2009 the FDA required the company that owns it to do a trial in which some patients got the drug and others got dacarbazine. This was both absurd and unethical. In a *New York Times* article about the drug, some doctors expressed concern about doing this, but they were going along with it nonetheless.

I can tell you one thing: no one working in the field who had this disease or had a family member with this disease would have allowed himself or his loved one to be randomized to the dacarbazine control arm. I sure wouldn't have.

In good conscience, you would have to say to the patient, "In my experience, dacarbazine almost never works and has bad side effects, but PLX4032 has been showing excellent and useful responses with minimal side effects. Is it okay with you if we give you dacarbazine?" I think I know what the answer would be.

Why was the FDA doing this? Because, according to the FDA, we needed to show that using PLX4032 increases survival compared with dacarbazine. That's nonsense. What we really needed to figure out was how to make these quality responses from PLX4032 permanent. I can think of a number of ways to do this, but none of them involve comparing PLX4032 alone with dacarbazine. Patients should have refused to enter the control arm, and doctors should have refused to offer it. In my view, every patient with metastatic melanoma in the country who had exhausted all reasonable therapeutic options should have had access to PLX4032.

After two years, an international study involving almost a thousand patients and costing $100 million showed results that were so positive for the new drug, now called vemurafenib, that the study was stopped. The FDA approved vemurafenib for use in metastatic melanoma in August 2011. How many patients lost time, or their lives, in the meantime?

The FDA has also failed to recognize a critical point that is unique to developing new cancer drugs: the patients waiting for these drugs are dying. In this sense, cancer is different from diabetes or hypertension or arthritis, where patients live with their diseases for a normal or near-normal life span. New drugs for these diseases need to be safe enough to be given over the normal lifetime of the patient.

By contrast, cancer drugs are tested first in people who have, on the average, six to twelve months to live, like those patients with metastatic melanoma I mentioned before. The drugs need to either kill cancer cells or stop them from growing over a relatively short period of time measured in months, not years. There is urgency in the cancer field not present in other fields. And if a drug works to some degree, the same population of patients wants and needs access to it long before the creaky approval process allows. The FDA refuses to acknowledge this.

The definition of effectiveness is in the eye of the beholder, and the beholder of record in the drug approval process is now an often inexperienced, overzealous, and overworked FDA reviewer afflicted with Frances Kelsey syndrome.

All of this could have been avoided. The framers of the cancer act were so aware of the potential FDA problem that the first Senate version of the cancer act included a provision to remove the NCI and cancer drug development from the control of the FDA. Authority for approval of new cancer drugs was to reside with the NCI, where a large cancer drug development program already existed, staffed with many experienced cancer doctors. This caused so much consternation among the regulatory community that at the urging of Ted Kennedy, who sponsored the original Senate bill for the cancer act, a ruinous compromise was negotiated between Benno Schmidt, the chairman of the Yarborough committee that framed the cancer act, and "Mr. Health," Representative Paul Rogers from Florida, the chairman of the Subcommittee on Health and the Environment of the House of Representatives. Among other things, it left the relationship between the NCI and the FDA intact.

But the advocates for rapid approval were right. Letting the NCI oversee things might not have been ideal, but it would have been better than what has happened and might have served as a model for the regulation of all new drugs outside the cancer field.

When I think about the FDA these days, I can't help but think about my friend Lee, whom I introduced earlier in the book. By 2008, twelve years after being diagnosed with advanced prostate cancer, he was failing and we'd run out of options for chemotherapy. Fortuitously, in July of that year, the *Journal of Clinical Oncology* paper about abiraterone was published.[3] Abiraterone inhibited a key enzyme, CYP17, involved in the body's manufacture of the male hormone testosterone. If you can't make testosterone, it can't drive your tumor's growth. This was another way of getting at the prostate cancer cell. I thought it might work for Lee.

The article was based only on a phase I study, but even so, the authors had reported an impressive response rate. And since we'd been using androgen deprivation for decades, it was unlikely we'd encounter any surprises with regard to side effects. As you may recall, I tried to get access to it for Lee but couldn't. A new trial had begun examining the effects of abiraterone in patients who were not as hormone resistant as those originally studied. But no provisions had been made by the FDA to provide drugs for patients with more advanced disease like those initially studied—like Lee. And no one was able to use it off study without getting into deep trouble with the FDA and the company that made the drug. It was a horrible state of affairs for patients operating, like Lee, on a slim margin—still alive, still wanting a chance, still capable of responding to therapy.

Although it involves horrendous paperwork and is time-consuming, a willing physician and patient can sometimes get drugs under a compassionate Investigational New Drug (IND) application, if the pharmaceutical company agrees to supply the drug and the FDA agrees to approve it. But over the years, the FDA has developed strict criteria as to what kind of patient is eligible and what kinds of drugs can be accessed this way. These paper criteria unfortunately trump the experience of the cancer doctor at the bedside. Lee's new doctor offered to try to get access to abiraterone under a compassionate IND, but his attempts failed.

Ironically, the major players in organized oncology—the NCI's clinical cooperative groups and its investigators and the American Society of Clinical Oncology, a society that prides itself on speaking on behalf of cancer patients—have also discouraged early access to drugs. They say they do so because early access is detrimental to the health of the NCI's clinical trials program, presumably because patients who access a new drug under a compassionate IND won't be available for clinical trials. But the patients who needed abiraterone and drugs like it were not even eligible for the new clinical trials. This has more to do with control than with reason.

In 2003, the Abigail Alliance for Better Access to Developmental Drugs filed suit against the FDA for denying access to new drugs to cancer patients.[4] The Abigail Alliance is named after the daughter of its founder, Frank Burroughs, who died of head and neck cancer. She was denied access to Erbitux, a drug I worked with while I was on the board of the ImClone company, which might, at least, have extended her life. The company itself had been more than willing to make the drug available free of charge, contending that it was a constitutional right of patients to have access to drugs even while still in development. The Abigail Alliance fights for the right of cancer patients to gain access to new cancer drugs. It's a good cause, and the organization's record is also a good one. So far, almost all of the drugs it has identified for early access have gone on to be FDA approved for cancer patients, although often many years later. Erbitux later showed impressive results in the treatment of head and neck cancers similar to Abigail's and has now been approved for that use by the FDA—too late for Abigail.

In its suit, the Abigail Alliance asserted that "a terminally ill patient, with no approved treatment options, has a right to decide for himself, in consultation with his own doctor, whether to take a drug the FDA concedes is safe and promising enough to be tested in substantial numbers of human subjects."

A three-judge panel of the U.S. Court of Appeals for the District of Columbia heard the case and found in the alliance's favor, based on the Fifth Amendment right to life.

The FDA requested that the D.C. Court of Appeals rehear the case. The Abigail Alliance contacted me and asked that I write an amicus curiae (meaning "friend of the court" brief) supporting its position. I declined because at the time I was writing a monthly editorial for the journal *Nature Reviews Clinical Oncology*, where I often took on issues related to the FDA. I was often critical of the agency, but sometimes I wrote in support of the FDA. I knew the FDA read my columns because whenever I said something nice I got a thank-you e-mail from the FDA commissioner, Andy von Eschenbach. I thought I should remain neutral, although I told Burroughs I supported his group's main mission.

That was a mistake on my part, because the American Society of Clinical Oncology agreed to write an amicus brief in support of the government. The gist of its brief was that open access to drugs under development would damage the clinical trials program of the NCI. It supplied no good data to support its position. In fact, there is plenty of evidence that this argument, often used by academics, is spurious.

In March 2007, the D.C. Court of Appeals this time sided with the FDA in an en banc vote of 8–2 ("en banc" means that this time the case was heard and voted on by the entire court of appeals). The amicus brief of a society that purports to speak on behalf of cancer patients had turned the tide against them. The Abigail Alliance appealed to the Supreme Court, but in January 2008 the Supreme Court declined to hear the case and let the opinion of the lower court stand.

I wasn't entirely surprised, because I'd been through this kind of thing before.

In the late 1970s, when I was director of the NCI's Division of Cancer Treatment, we actually solved this problem and provided access to new and potentially useful cancer drugs under the NCI's jurisdiction if they began to show clinical benefit. The FDA didn't like this. The group leader for oncologic drugs, a man by the name of R.S.K. Young, tried to stop it—and all of cancer drug development to boot.

Young's boss, Dr. Richard Crout, head of the Bureau of Drugs, was sympathetic to what we were doing but felt hamstrung by his staff's link to Congress—especially the FDA's champion Ted Kennedy—and he was afraid of appearing soft on cancer drugs if Kennedy got wind of what we were up to. I was frustrated by what I saw as weak FDA leadership—allowing a single mid-level staffer to hold up all of cancer drug development.

Ironically, I had helped to train Young. He had come to the NCI as a clinical associate in the early 1970s, when I was chief of the solid tumor service of the NCI's medicine branch. He was a nice-looking, Chinese American doctor with jet-black hair—very serious and quiet. He had gotten both his M.D. and his Ph.D. in pharmacology at Yale's medical school and cancer drug pharmacology program, so his credentials were impeccable. He was a good doctor and bright enough that I asked him to stay on and work with us in the lab. Ultimately, I dangled the possibility of one of the coveted slots as a senior investigator on our service. We were already heavily involved in the curative treatments of lymphomas, and these were much-sought-after jobs. Young opted instead to work with Robert Gallo in the Laboratory of Tumor Cell Biology—which was an exciting job, too. Or it should have been.

Gallo would go on to be the developer of the diagnostic test for the AIDS virus that saved many lives and the co-discoverer of the virus that causes AIDS. He also discovered T cell growth factor, later named interleukin-2, an important component of the immunotherapy programs developed by Steve Rosenberg. At this point, AIDS hadn't been discovered yet, but Gallo, a brilliant, charming, and volatile scientist, had an active lab program searching for cancer viruses. Positions in his program were actively sought by the associates.

Not long after Young went over there, Gallo called me. "Vince," he said, "what's with this guy?" Apparently, he had offered Young the opportunity to work on an exciting problem related to a new cancer virus, but Young's preference was to manage Bob's many research contracts. This was the work of an administrator, not a scientist, who usually avoided these tasks like poison. Also, Young declined Bob's offer to stay for a third year in favor of going to work for the FDA to review drug applications. I was dumbfounded. It was unusual for someone as well trained as R.S.K. Young to make such a choice. I called Young one more time and offered him a position on our service, but he immediately said no. And off he went to the FDA.

I forgot about him until he emerged about five years later as the group leader for oncologic drugs, the unit responsible for the review and approval of anticancer drugs, and virtually shut us down. He told me he didn't believe in the usefulness of cancer drugs and meant to stop their development. It was during this time that I went public at the Division of Cancer Treatment's scientific advisory board. I invited Young to a board meeting to explain his position. By law, these meetings are open to the public and covered by the press, so his performance was well recorded and created quite a stir.

He told the board what he had told me and then, picking up a thick copy of the Code of Federal Regulations he had brought with him, he waved it in the air and said to the board, "This is the bible—this is the bible." Like most of his current counterparts, he appeared to be obsessed with FDA regulations.

As reported in *The Cancer Letter* on November 14, 1975, after the meeting, Young admitted that the delays were based on form rather than substance. He said the decision to enforce previously overlooked regulatory details had been made following a recent wave of criticism that the agency had been negligent—or worse—in approving certain drugs. Young mentioned the scandal in which the army was permitted to test LSD and referred to criticism aired at hearings conducted by Senator Edward Kennedy's Health Subcommittee. This made no sense. LSD had nothing in common with cancer drugs for dying patients. We all wondered what was driving Young to do this. He was a smart man, a concert-level pianist who got his law degree at night while at the FDA. My feeling is that it was a compulsion with him. Even when they defied logic, he preferred regulations. There was nothing we could do to change him.

I appealed to the FDA commissioner, who wouldn't give me any support. So I turned to the head of the FDA's Bureau of Drugs—Dick Crout. In many meetings over the following weeks, we tried to come up with a way around Young's tactics. We solved the problem by developing a master plan for cancer drug development that, after months of tedious work, we submitted to the Bureau of Drugs for approval. The master plan was to govern how we dealt with all cancer drugs, including access to them by needy patients.

But Young persisted in blocking cancer drug approval. As part of his paralyzing tactics, he held up the approval of the drug cisplatin for three years, even though every cancer doctor in the country knew it was an effective agent and very useful in testicular cancer. He did this by testifying before the ODAC, the Oncologic Drugs Advisory Committee—in an unofficial capacity during his lunch break, as a "concerned citizen"—because most of the studies involved using cisplatin in combination with other drugs. Experienced investigators, following their instincts, had skipped trying the drug alone, because they knew it worked best as part of a cocktail of drugs, just as we had found in treating many other kinds of cancers. Fearing the FDA would approve this practice, he testified before the ODAC to protest his agency's own positions. (He told me in a recent phone call that had he testified as an FDA employee, he would have had to support its position.)

Young wanted data on cisplatin tested alone in testicular cancer and in a randomized controlled trial against other treatments, as required in the Code of Federal Regulations, his bible. Our data in childhood leukemia and Hodgkin's disease had already shown the need for drugs to be used in combination to cure cancers. What Young wanted to do—treating patients with a single agent, cisplatin—would have meant jeopardizing the lives of patients. (When cisplatin was ultimately approved, it proved part of the curative combination chemotherapy treatment for Lance Armstrong, who had very advanced metastatic testicular cancer in his lungs and even in his brain.) It was after this that my staff dubbed R.S.K. Young "Risky" Young. The failure to use cisplatin in combination for testicular cancer could cost people their lives.

To my mind, what Young was doing was the beginning of the FDA's foray into regulating research and practice. Young was the forerunner of Richard Pazdur; both were cut from the same cloth—either that or the air pumped into the FDA building has some kind of pro-regulatory gas in it.

A couple of years later, I was asked by the Bristol-Myers Squibb company if I would support the extension of its cisplatin patent for three years as compensation for the unwarranted delay in the approval of the drug. I agreed and along with my former deputy director of DCT, Steve Carter, who was now a vice president of global drug development for Bristol-Myers Squibb, met with Margaret Heckler, Reagan's secretary of health and human services, and the assistant secretary, Ed Brandt, to make the case. Heckler approved our request for a three-year extension. In return, Bristol-Myers Squibb supported $30 million a year of research for three years at the NCI. Cisplatin went on to become one of the most useful cancer drugs ever developed, and several other platinum-related drugs have also been developed— one of which was used effectively on my friend Lee.

We did have one period of relative calm with the FDA, when, after a brief stint by interim director Jere Goyan, Arthur Hull Hayes became commissioner in 1981. Within weeks of his appointment, I made the case for the removal of Young from any involvement in cancer drug development. Hayes had Young transferred to the section on cardio-vascular drugs. Unfortunately, Hayes lasted only two years. He ran afoul of longtime FDA staffers.

The master plan we created addressed the issue of poor access to drugs by putting experimental drugs in one of three categories la-beled Groups A, B, and C.

In keeping with FDA requirements, Group A and B drugs were distributed only to the investigators involved in early phase I and II trials. But if a drug in Groups A and B showed clinical benefit in more than one trial, we would put it into a separate group, Group C, where regardless of its stage of development, it could be made available to the patients with tumor types for which benefit had been shown.

This whole system came to be known as the Group C drug distri-bution system. Any physician who had filed a Form 1572 (a one-page registration form the FDA uses to keep track of clinical investigators) could access a drug for an individual patient if, in his or her judg-ment, it was appropriate for that patient.

The determination of a drug's entry into Group C was made by NCI physicians, and the determination that the drug might be bene-ficial to an individual patient was made by the patient's doctor at the bedside—not by FDA bureaucrats. And the NCI took the responsi-bility for acquiring, tracking, and distributing the drugs to physicians and patients; there were minimal reporting requirements for the pa-tient's physician (only serious adverse effects needed to be reported).

The FDA staff, especially Young, disliked this system, but they were stuck with it. And it worked. During its existence, more than twenty anticancer drugs were categorized as Group C and made available to cancer patients who needed them. The pharmaceutical companies were willing to supply the drugs for free because they saw the NCI's designation of their drugs into Group C as a step toward ultimate acceptance. Physicians saw it as another treatment option for their patients.

No harm was done to the NCI's clinical trials program, either. I know, because I was running it. The clinical cooperative groups recruited more, not fewer, patients into clinical trials. Increasing awareness of the usefulness of cancer drugs made it more acceptable for patients to enter these studies.

But nothing fails like success. The NCI's drug distribution system had not been codified into the federal regulations by the FDA, nor had it been mandated by Congress. The FDA unilaterally suspended the NCI's Group C program toward the end of my time as the NCI director in 1987, when the Investigational New Drug treatment regulations were passed in response to the demands of AIDS patients for access to new drugs (again Congress acted at the behest of the FDA). Treatment INDs were individual protocols for a drug that could be approved by the FDA and used to provide access to a new drug for AIDS patients. Instead of adopting the Group C mechanism for AIDS patients, the FDA lumped cancer patients in with AIDS patients. The NCI's system was dumped in favor of the new system of treatment INDs.

Ironically, treatment INDs worked for AIDS patients because with so few drugs available at the time, one treatment IND could be developed and used at multiple centers. For cancer patients, with a hundred different types of cancers and many more drug choices, the treatment IND has been a failure. It has made access to cancer drugs very restricted, which is where we find ourselves today.

The treatment IND was further modified in the Food and Drug Administration Modernization Act of 1997. The bill required that the FDA's staff—rather than the NCI and cancer doctors—determine if a drug was both safe and effective enough for distribution to a particular patient, a patient who, of course, they had never seen. And the FDA's staff was to determine *specifically* (now a requirement in law) that such distribution would not have an adverse effect on clinical trials. Of course, the policy merely perpetuated a myth. There was no way to determine this except by asking those who were conducting clinical trials, and those conducting the trials always say yes as a means of protecting their turf.

The FDA Modernization Act also required that the sponsor of the drug for a treatment IND submit enough information to meet the requirements of an FDA IND. No busy physician can afford the time or has the support to develop individual treatment INDs.

Lee's doctor even tried but was discouraged from doing it because of the potential adverse effect on the ongoing clinical trial of abiraterone.

It was around the time that we submitted the master plan to the FDA's Bureau of Drugs that the FDA established the ODAC. I mentioned it earlier as the committee Young approached to make his case against cisplatin. It first met in September 1978, during the tenure of the FDA commissioner Don Kennedy, partly to address the criticism the NCI often leveled at the FDA that it did not have enough experience with cancer drugs to be making these decisions by itself.

The ODAC is purely advisory. It has no real authority, not even to request that the FDA ask its advice on a specific drug. And it hasn't worked. Committees are never a substitute for experience.

The ODAC's mission includes the review of selected New Drug Applications as well as the status of old drugs that the FDA might be considering for removal from the marketplace. But again, the ODAC's reviews are limited to those drugs the FDA chooses to present to it. And while its makeup has changed over the years, its members are selected by the FDA commissioner or his designee. It can also include one technically qualified person recommended by consumer organizations, and recently a nonvoting membership has been given to a person who represents the interests of industry. But the FDA stacks the ODAC with as many people of like mind as it can. There are no critics of the FDA on the ODAC. Freireich has been nominated many times by individuals and organizations. The FDA knows it would set off an outcry were it to disapprove his nomination, so what it does is this: it places Freireich on standby status. He has never been called to serve.

The ODAC meets only four times a year. Meetings are covered under the committee practices act, which requires that meetings of any group of outside consultants be open to the public.[5] As a consequence, these meetings have become a bit of a circus. Advocates show up wearing T-shirts emblazoned with the name of the drug they want approved. They wave placards. That happened at one ODAC meeting when the prostate cancer vaccine Provenge was under discussion.[6]

The meetings are governed by rigid formats. The principal investigator of a drug under consideration, often someone from the pharmaceutical industry, presents the data on the drug. The FDA staffer leading the review presents the FDA's position on the drug, and Richard Pazdur presents his point of view. Then the committee is asked to vote on a series of questions offered by the FDA. The FDA likes to boast that it rarely goes against the recommendations of the ODAC, but the ODAC only votes on the FDA's positions.

Right from the start, the ODAC has been a setup, beginning with Young's appearance before it as a "concerned citizen," despite the fact that he was also the official controlling the approval process.

In the late 1970s and early 1980s, the ODAC became the playground of a prominent oncologist, Charles "Chuck" Moertel, a good friend of mine, although we disagreed about almost everything having to do with the development of new treatments.

It was Moertel who convinced the FDA to use survival as an end point for new drug approval—much to the consternation of the oncology community, for reasons I will outline for you in a moment.

Moertel was an archconservative when it came to drug testing. He was at the Mayo Clinic in Rochester, Minnesota, and because of the nature of its referral pattern (patients came from a distance, stayed a few days, and returned at six-week intervals), he designed his drug schedules accordingly. Moertel's specialty was colon cancer. He began to work with a promising drug for colorectal cancer called 5-fluorouracil (5-FU), but it never worked for his patients. The reason seemed simple to me. Unless you believed in magic, you couldn't treat actively growing cancer cells on an every-six-weeks schedule. Doing so meant ignoring everything we knew about the biology of tumor growth. It is interesting to note that after everyone abandoned Moertel's weird scheduling practices, 5-FU went on to become a proven drug in colorectal cancers and is now part of every effective treatment regimen used around the world. But Moertel and the FDA set the drug and the approval process back two decades. No wonder the FDA loved him.

The FDA quickly exploited the breach in the oncologic community, and Moertel became a fixture on the ODAC. With urging from the FDA, he made the case that the only acceptable end point for approval of a new drug, what needed to be demonstrated, was that the new drug would improve chances for survival compared with existing treatment. Defying logic, all ODAC members went along with him.

The bottom line is that the ODAC is a board like any other advisory board, and there is a peculiarity of boards and committees that can explain their sometimes illogical behavior. It involves a psychological characteristic first noted at the turn of the twentieth century in *The Crowd* by Gustave Le Bon, a French psychiatrist.[7] Of the crowd, Le Bon wrote, "Under certain given circumstances . . . an agglomeration of men presents new characteristics very different from those of the individuals composing it . . . A collective mind is formed, doubtless transitory, but presenting very clearly defined characteristics." This collective mind makes individuals "feel, think, and act in a manner quite different from that in which each individual of them would feel, think, and act were he in a state of isolation." The new behavior, he says, does not consist of an averaging of the individual parts but rather a new entity, and often, an illogical one. Psychological crowds, according to Le Bon (Le Bon's definition of a crowd ranged from a few to thousands of people), are affected by suggestion, and suggestion leads to contagion. Le Bon's astute observation anticipated the effect of demagogues such as Adolf Hitler on the behavior of large crowds.

It is interesting to sit at board and committee meetings with Le Bon's ideas in mind. The ODAC is the best example I know of a psychological crowd, comprising individuals who privately will tell you one thing but collectively will do another.

So, why the controversy over the FDA using *survival* as an end point? The cancer cell that has been exposed to multiple drug treatments is one wily beast. If you grow cancer cells in a petri dish and put in a good concentration of a drug, something equivalent to what you would use in the clinic, it will kill most of them. But those that survive will grow back and be resistant to that drug, at least in the doses that you used. If you increase the dose, the same thing will happen. It will kill most of the cells, but those that survive will grow back resistant to the bigger dose. The only way you can circumvent this is to give huge doses, amounts way out of line with what would be tolerable in a human being. Barring that, the cells will be resistant to any dose you can give. If you now do the same thing to those cells with another drug, you can make the cancer cells in the petri dish resistant to both drugs and a third one, too. And something else happens. Cancer cells will begin to develop resistance to drugs they have never seen by ramping up a mechanism that can pump most foreign chemicals out of the cell. The gene that controls this is known as the MDR gene, for multidrug resistance. The result is that even if you now expose the cancer cells to a new drug, you won't kill many of them at all.

This is what happens to cancer patients like Lee. After several drug treatments, their cells have become too smart to respond to anything, at least in the doses you can give without causing too much damage to the rest of the body.

So new drugs face a huge hurdle when tested in patients with very advanced, heavily pretreated disease. You can easily miss a significant benefit in this population of patients. Frankly, it is a bit of a miracle that we actually spot any activity in response to a new drug under these circumstances. That's why I am always very impressed when any new drug produces complete remissions in patients with advanced disease. When that happens, you can bet the drug will eventually turn out to be useful. But those at the FDA rarely use that kind of information to move a drug forward. Instead, like my friend Chuck Moertel, they would prefer that a new drug improve survival when compared with an old drug.

It is unrealistic to use survival as an end point. Consider the number of cancer cells a drug has to kill to be effective. The average patient with advanced cancer has more than a kilogram of tumor on board. That's many billions of cancer cells, because a lump about one centimeter across contains roughly one billion cells. Even after surgery, when a primary cancer has been removed and no errant cells can be detected, a patient can have more than a billion cancer cells circulating around the body.

To see a complete response to treatment, a drug has to kill 99.99 percent of the cancer cells. And then a very curious thing happens.

The time it takes for the surviving tumor cells to grow back to their pretreatment levels varies depending on the number of cells that have survived the treatment. Smaller populations grow back faster than larger populations. It seems counterintuitive, but it's true. The net effect is that if you have two treatments—one that reduces the cancer cell population in a patient to just a few cells, and one that reduces the population to one billion cells—neither patient will have visible tumor masses at that point. But after five years, both will have the same number of cancer cells present, as the rapidly growing smaller population catches up. The five-year survival rates will be the same. But the treatment that reduced the population to a few cells is the one you want to go forward with. But which one is that? You cannot tell by using five-year survival rates as an end point.

This is called the Norton-Simon effect, named after two of my colleagues who discovered it. This alone should lead to the reconsideration of the use of survival rates in advanced cancer patients as a requirement for approval of a new drug.

When you combine multidrug resistance and the Norton-Simon effect, the deck is stacked against any new drug. If the crude end point we look for is survival, it is not surprising that many new drugs seem ineffective. We need new ways to test new drugs in cancer patients, ways that allow testing at earlier stages of disease, but investigators are afraid to suggest this for fear that the FDA and its human investigations committees will disapprove.

To be fair, the FDA has approved cancer drugs based only on response, or more often on progression-free survival, but this is not its preference. Unless investigators go head-to-head with the FDA when they design their protocols, the FDA will gravitate to using survival as the primary end point.

On many occasions, I have seen doctors, especially in the pharmaceutical industry, flinch at the suggestion that they argue with the FDA to get a more realistic end point; they fear the enmity of the FDA. Flinching may cost their company many millions of dollars in unnecessary clinical studies, and it may cost cancer patients access to important, alternative treatments. As we've seen, that's what happened with the thousand-patient, $100 million study comparing the exciting vemurafenib to the useless dacarbazine.

But the biggest problem we have, one I discussed at the beginning of this chapter, is that the FDA now routinely regulates research and practice. In doing so, it has become the oncologist of last resort.

Drugs are now approved not for a specific cancer or for general use in a variety of cancers but for a specific *stage* of a specific cancer and specifically after and only after patients have had all current treatments, which are listed drug by drug, and the treatments have all failed. Doctors risk FDA censure if they use an approved drug under any other circumstance, and patients are penalized because insurance companies won't pay for treatments not approved by the FDA.

The vital insight gained by using an approved drug in a different way for a different tumor has been lost.

Researchers need to get FDA approval for each and every variation they wish to study, including midcourse corrections in studies. Because the FDA requires it, institutional review boards (IRBs) require it, and this has created a vicious cycle of review and rereview. Because it can take as long as, in one case, eight hundred days from the birth of an idea to the inception of a clinical study, you can see the problem.[8]

And the people who are reviewing this research are not the ones trained to do it. This has had a stultifying effect on clinical research and has turned the NCI's clinical trials program into a muddy morass. The most innovative studies are the first to go. Le Bon's psychological crowd effect is running rampant with the review process, becoming an end in itself.

I'd like to be able to say that as cancer drugs have become increasingly more complex and sophisticated, the FDA has as well. But it has not.

Many of the new cancer drugs, for instance, such as the monoclonal antibodies Herceptin and Erbitux, or the new kinase inhibitors, such as vemurafenib, attack very specific targets, but many have little activity when used alone. They work by *enhancing* the action of other drugs, usually by resetting the cell death mechanism the cancer cell has cleverly deactivated. They work better in combination with other drugs, and these combinations of drugs represent some of the most exciting advances in cancer chemotherapy.

The FDA still requires that they be tested one at a time to observe the side effects of each one alone. This is fine, but it is the requirement of efficacy that is now a problem.

We are approaching what we might have considered nirvana years ago. We can design drugs that will hit a specific target, and by being so specific, they have fewer side effects. But because effective treatment almost always requires hitting more than one target at the same time, some very good and relatively safe cancer drugs show no evidence of effectiveness when used alone.

What a dilemma. After spending millions of dollars developing a drug, a company may be forced to abandon it for lack of efficacy, when, if approved, it would be another exciting tool for clinical investigators who want to explore combinations of targeted therapies in post-marketing research trials. Compound that with the FDA's insistence on testing them first on patients with very advanced, resistant disease, and many potentially useful drugs don't look so good. As a result, drug companies are reluctant to invest money in new cancer drugs, because they might never make it past the FDA's hurdles. People are dying not because drugs don't exist but because they can't get them.

You might recall that on September 11, 2010, precisely two years after Lee's death, I got an e-mail from Howard Scher at MSKCC telling me that there was a news release accompanying the completion of the study of abiraterone confirming the early results.[9] Patients on abiraterone were surviving so much longer that the study was unblinded and stopped early. The company that made abiraterone also announced an expanded access program to make the drug available to patients who needed it, though it was years away from FDA approval. Too late for Lee.

Four days later, at a ceremony at FDA headquarters to hand out the Frances Kelsey annual award marking the fiftieth anniversary of Kelsey's campaign against thalidomide, Janet Woodcock, director of the FDA's Center for Drug Evaluation and Research, said, "Without Kelsey's efforts, we would not have the drug regulations we have today."

Kelsey, who had retired from the FDA at the extraordinary age of ninety and was now ninety-six years old, listened from a wheelchair and then spoke a few words of thanks to an overflow crowd.

9

I had come to the NCI a reluctant physician, determined to put in my two years and leave, hopefully untainted by my foray into that hopeless field. Instead, I'd stayed nearly three decades and found my life's work and my own version of Freireich's evangelism.

Mine was of a slightly different variety from Freireich's. There was my research, and there were my patients, who continued to be my motivation. But there was also the challenge of organizing the growing infrastructure of cancer so that patients actually benefited from it.

When the war on cancer was being formulated, there were only three centers outside the NCI that specialized in cancer. One aim of the National Cancer Act was to provide patients with better access to new therapies by creating new cancer centers. The act called for at least fifteen more centers to be built as quickly as possible and, ultimately, for every state to have a comprehensive cancer center.

The vision for the new centers was that they would be miniversions of the NCI, each serving a defined geographic area and able to deal with, and take responsibility for, cancer in its area. They were expected to be involved in the entire gamut of research, from cause and prevention to diagnosis, treatment, and rehabilitation. They were to be places where results from the laboratory could quickly be applied in the clinic to help cancer patients, places where new approaches to diagnosis and treatment would be developed. They were envisioned as hotbeds of translational research, also known as bench-to-bedside research, where teams of physicians and scientists could gather with the freedom to think their way through the cancer problem.

In leaving the NCI, I was going out into the real world of cancer care—where the rubber met the road, so to speak. I knew the numbers. Eighty percent of all cancer patients were cared for in the community by private physicians. Only 20 percent went to one of the NCI cancer centers. I knew what we knew at this point about cancer: it is a genetic disease caused by a breakdown of genes responsible for growth, and we now knew what those genes were and how they worked. I knew where we were and what we could do for patients.

But how well was this being translated to patients?

Over the next two decades, I would see how the war on cancer was faring, first as physician in chief at Memorial Sloan Kettering Cancer Center, the largest private cancer center in the world, and then at Yale Cancer Center, one of the major cancer centers created by the National Cancer Act.

Memorial Sloan Kettering was founded in 1884 as the New York Cancer Hospital.

Fifteen years later, its name was changed to General Memorial Hospital for Cancer and Allied Diseases. In 1945, Alfred Sloan, chairman of General Motors and a trustee of Memorial Hospital, and Charles Kettering, vice president and director of research for GM, arranged a $4 million gift from GM. The gift was to establish a research arm of Memorial Hospital, and it would be called the Sloan Kettering Institute. For the next two decades, then, the combined hospital and lab would be known as Memorial Sloan Kettering Institute.

In 1971, when the National Cancer Act was passed, Memorial Sloan Kettering Institute, one of the three hospitals devoted to cancer in the United States, was deemed a role model for what all newly constructed centers should strive to be. Indeed, after the cancer act was passed, the NCI designated Memorial Sloan Kettering Institute a national cancer center without further review. That would change the hospital's name once again. Now it would be Memorial Sloan Kettering Cancer Center.

It was a seal of approval of sorts, a nod to the fact that the center offered one-stop shopping for anyone in the New York area who needed cancer care, though it wasn't just the locals who availed themselves of it. In 1988, when I arrived at MSKCC, as it is often abbreviated, the center was seeing more patients than any other cancer center in the country.

Because it was a private institution, a board of managers collectively worth about $10 billion ran it. When I got there, Benno Schmidt was just turning over the chairmanship of the board to James D. Robinson III, the chairman and CEO of American Express, whom everyone referred to as Jimmy Three Sticks. (He hated the name.)

Other board members included Laurance Rockefeller and a group of wealthy, powerful people, assembled by him along with the Rockefeller family, including Richard Gelb, CEO of Bristol-Myers Squibb; Ben Rosen, chairman of Compaq computer; Lou Gerstner, vice-chair of American Express; and John Reed, chair and CEO of Citicorp.

Laurance Rockefeller, who was rumored to be worth $5 billion, had been in the habit of writing a check at the end of the year to cover any MSKCC deficits, which were usually in the range of $10 million.

Soon after I arrived, Paul Marks, the president of MSKCC and the person who had recruited me for the job of physician in chief, pulled me aside and said, "Vince, you have to understand that Laurance owns this place. What Laurance wants Laurance gets." Laurance's most recent desire had been to create a new laboratory building across the street from Sloan Kettering, on Sixty-Seventh Street, which he had contributed $35 million for and named after his father.

The place seemed to have an endless supply of money. The board regularly raised about $85 million a year from philanthropy, far outstripping any other cancer center in the country at that time. MSKCC also had an endowment worth about $800 million—more than most universities in the country.

Because of the institute's size and history, and the reach and power of the board, many of the world's wealthiest people flew to New York City for their care. About 6 percent of admissions came from overseas. They paid their bills in cash.

MSKCC, in short, had all the money it needed to be a top-notch center. And the board believed it was. At every board meeting, Jimmy Robinson liked to intone that he demanded the highest quality at American Express and he expected no less at MSKCC. But the truth was that while MSKCC had the potential to be the best cancer center in the world, it wasn't.

The benefit of being a large, freestanding center (meaning not embedded in a university, as later ones were) such as MSKCC is its freedom from teaching responsibilities, and it is full of doctors who specialize in any given cancer. If you have lung cancer, for example, a center like MSKCC may have as many as five doctors within each specialty dedicated to it—five oncologists, five surgeons, five radiologists. That's a lot. And because these institutes are large, they see every permutation of tumors. This experience is a huge strength.

The downside is that the center can get locked into one approach to a disease or become dominated by one specialty. All three of the freestanding cancer centers in 1971—MSKCC, MD Anderson in Houston, Texas, and Roswell Park in Buffalo, New York—were dominated by surgeons.

Among MSKCC's weaknesses were a failure to keep up with new advances, a tendency to allow the old guard to reflexively reject novel approaches, and the long-standing bugaboo that has always dogged cancer—a tendency to value lab research for its own sake, rather than to see research as a way to advance care for patients.

Shortly after I arrived, the board asked me to do a complete institutional evaluation and to create a five-year plan for improvement.

Over the next several months, I evaluated every department and every person in every department. While it was supposed to be kept private, all the staff knew I was doing this, and it created a lot of anxiety. Every time I saw the chief of surgery socially, he would sidle up to me and say, "Vince, I am part of the solution, not part of the problem."

MSKCC had some strengths. For instance, it had, in the person of Murray Brennan, one of the best cancer surgeons in the country. Brennan had come to MSKCC from Steve Rosenberg's branch at the NCI, where his research interest had been sarcomas. He was such a good surgeon that he loved to operate; Murray would operate on anything. If he was in the hospital and a case of appendicitis came in, he would do the surgery.

He felt strongly that the chief had to be a jack-of-all-trades, able to do anything. And he was technically so good that he could get away with it. I actually used to scrub in with him just to watch him work.

Murray had wound up with a lot of GI cases at MSKCC and had become one of the most skillful gastrointestinal cancer surgeons in the country. He had learned to do research with Steve, which made him part of an unusual breed—surgeons who do research. Steve was one. Bernie Fisher was another. Murray had a lab at MSKCC, but Paul Marks didn't think much of it. He referred to the lab as Brennan's sandbox, meaning he considered it more of an amusement for Murray than a productive lab.

But other departments weren't in good shape. If you weren't a surgeon or a radiotherapist, your home was in the big sprawling department of medicine, where the doctors treated mostly advanced cancers with drugs. The department of medicine had fallen behind the times and needed reorganization. It was full of fiefdoms of old-guard physicians mostly interested in defending their own turf. There was very little collaboration within departments and virtually none across departments.

Its breast cancer program, for example, barely existed. Here was an example of the old guard keeping out new approaches. In 1988, lumpectomy was a clear option for patients with small breast tumors. But every woman with breast cancer who went to MSKCC still got a radical mastectomy. That's because the old guard at this hospital—which to many was the epitome of topflight cancer care in the United States—had stubbornly resisted the lumpectomy and adjuvant care.

Ten years earlier, when the research supporting lumpectomy was coming to light, I'd gone to the auditorium of Rockefeller University, across the street from MSKCC, to listen to a lecture delivered by Bernie Fisher, the surgeon who, you'll recall, led the studies that demonstrated the effectiveness of lumpectomy.

As Bernie stood at the podium, presenting his data, with his slides projected on the screen behind him, Jerry Urban, chief of breast surgery at MSKCC, had risen from his seat and proceeded to scream at Bernie in front of the audience of five hundred or so doctors. "You're a traitor to your own profession," he'd shouted. "What you are saying is pure nonsense. Until we know more, every woman with breast cancer should receive a radical mastectomy"—ignoring the fact that if all women got radical mastectomies, there would be no way to know more and to compare results of a less invasive operation.

Urban had a lot of clout, and he was the go-to guy anytime someone rich and powerful had breast cancer, including Happy Rockefeller and Betty Ford.

At the time of Bernie's lecture, Urban had just published his own data on the super-radical mastectomy, a brutal, disfiguring procedure in which, as I have said, the surgeon would remove the breast, the axillary nodes, the chest muscles, and the internal mammary lymph nodes all in a single procedure. In terms of treatment, Fisher and Urban were dramatically opposed.

But Urban's data were sloppy. He did no comparative studies, merely operating and collecting his cases after the fact for publication. He selected cases in which women had earlier-stage disease, in which you'd expect a better outcome. And there was evidence from Bernie Fisher's lab work that breast cancer spread early into the bloodstream, which is why a radical mastectomy wasn't more effective than a lumpectomy. Urban didn't believe this and had instead developed the super-radical mastectomy, which ran counter to any intelligent thinking.

Bernie Fisher's findings were based on good science. But that didn't spare him the rage of his peers, who weren't ready to let go of the old way of doing things. One after another, members of the audience, esteemed surgeons, many of them, stood up and screamed, echoing Jerry Urban. I was shocked by the vitriol.

Bernie simply waited for the diatribe to end. Then he calmly asked for his last slide. It showed two curves stretched out over time, one a gently down-sloping convex curve with the label "PR." The other was a sharply up-sloping concave curve with the label "CR." The audience was perplexed. So was I. Being a medical oncologist, I wondered if "CR" stood for "complete remission" and "PR" meant "partial remission." But I couldn't figure out how that applied to surgery. After a minute or so of puzzled silence, Bernie dropped his bomb. "Here is the problem with my critics," he said as he pointed to the up-sloping curve with his laser pointer. "Increasing cerebral rigidity," he sang out, aiming his laser at "CR."

A gasp erupted from the audience, followed by a few angry murmurs. "And this," he said, moving his laser to the downward-sloping curve, "is matched by 'PR,' decreasing penile rigidity."

Now the anger in the audience was bubbling over. Voices grew louder; doctors were turning to each other in collective agreement that Bernie Fisher had gone too far.

But the clincher was his final statement. Fisher said his critics, in continuing to recommend the radical mastectomy, were mostly motivated by economic reasons. Put bluntly, he said, surgeons could charge more for a mastectomy than for the less invasive lumpectomy. At that, Jerry Urban and his colleague Guy Robbins walked out. Half of the audience followed them.

Bernie had won, if you counted solid data and a well-crafted parting shot as winning. But a decade later, patients at MSKCC were still losing, Urban and Robbins were still there, and while the standard of care was now a lumpectomy, MSKCC had quietly morphed over to the "modified radical mastectomy" without any testing to see if it was as good as or worse than the radical mastectomy. It took less tissue, but it wasn't a lumpectomy. And they had ensured that protocols involving the use of radiotherapy or chemotherapy with surgery had not been put in place. They just didn't sign on to any protocols that involved adjuvant chemotherapy, and without such patients no studies could proceed. Urban and Robbins were really private practitioners operating within the walls of a big cancer center.

They were operating on approximately fifteen hundred cases of breast cancer a year. But they didn't have a single adjuvant chemotherapy protocol to offer as a complement to surgery. And women had to be aware, on their own, that such options existed. If a woman needed or wanted adjuvant chemotherapy, she was referred elsewhere. Usually back to her primary physician. This was what was passing for "the very best."

MSKCC's lymphoma program was also marginal. In 1988, it was mostly either trying to prove that what someone else was doing wasn't good or modifying what someone else was doing so it could have an MSKCC study to call its own. There was no original thinking going on, no good use being made of a high volume of patients. The presiding attitude was still "If it wasn't invented at MSKCC, it couldn't be good," and yet MSKCC wasn't inventing anything significant. Its leukemia program was also not up-to-date. MSKCC was still using tired old programs. All the action in adult leukemia had shifted to its major competitor, the MD Anderson Cancer Center in Houston, where Jay Freireich was working.

The department of head and neck cancer was also lagging behind. The chief of the department, though technically skilled, refused to consider using more radiotherapy and chemotherapy, both of which had been shown to improve outcome in some patients with head and neck cancers.

The same was true for the highly curable testicular cancer. The standard had been developed at Indiana University's cancer center by

Larry Einhorn, but it was not in use at MSKCC, which was using a much more complicated treatment that was not as good but had been invented at MSKCC. But MSKCC's patients, many of whom were paying cash, out of pocket, weren't seeing these advances. And they didn't know it.

The tenure system was such that it was hard for new doctors to advance, and old ones, who should have made room for them, were disinclined to do so. In fact, some of the old guard needed to go. The nurses told me that one prominent, politically connected doctor made rounds in the evening after he'd been drinking. It was an open secret. But with his connections, he'd been left alone.

(Another prominent surgeon, also a heavy drinker, was known to imbibe until the wee hours of the morning. His colleagues wondered out loud if he was sober enough to operate at 7:00 a.m., when the first of the day's patients was wheeled into the operating room.)

Yet another outstanding surgeon had developed a creeping paralysis in his legs so disabling that he was unable to stand. He continued to operate sitting on a stool. It was only a matter of time before the paralysis would begin to affect his arms and hands. Most likely, the way we'd discover this would be an accident in surgery.

MSKCC's wealth, even the money donated by grateful patients, seemed to be relegated to labs. The new facility named for Rockefeller's father was quite lavish. But the researchers weren't doing much impressive work there. And the clinicians who wanted to do research weren't encouraged to pursue their work. The sandbox analogy applied to any clinician who tried to couple lab research with clinical medicine. There was very little conversation between the scientists at the Sloan Kettering Institute and the doctors at the hospital occupying the same New York City block.

Meanwhile, the patient care facilities were old and cramped, and patients waited on long lines for their care. The spaces were poor, too, with orange rugs worn and stained with coffee and blood. The radiotherapy department had fallen into disrepair. Its physical plant was archaic; its equipment, out-of-date.

With their wealthy clients, though—the ones who made donations—MSKCC had the deputy physician in chief greet them as they walked in the front door of the hospital on York Avenue. He walked them through the system, bypassing long lines and unsightly waiting rooms, and personally drew their blood samples.

At either end on each of the clinical floors were two private rooms reserved for the rich and powerful. When they were not available, a bed was removed from a double room, converting it to a private room, which decreased the number of available beds for other patients.

What all this meant for the general patient was depressing. I relayed my findings to the board, much to the displeasure of my boss, Paul Marks. He preferred to keep the technicalities of what was happening at the center at a distance from the board. In fact, he liked to brief me before board meetings about what I was and was not to relate during meetings. But the board members were expecting me to tell them the stark truth about what I'd found. They'd listened to what I said and agreed on changes.

We started holding "state-of-the-art" conferences on head and neck cancers and breast cancer. For six months, I asked the staff of all the departments to saturate the grand rounds and major conferences at the hospital with lectures on specific diseases.

I scheduled a special grand rounds in head and neck cancers to show that the results were better by far using chemotherapy and less destructive surgery, but the message fell on deaf ears.

In breast cancer, almost every conference we held for six months was given by an outside expert or recognized leader in the field. Each of them was asked to define what he or she saw as state of the art. The goal was to assemble our own state-of-the-art program from the best of what we heard.

In the case of breast cancer, of course, that meant inviting Bernie Fisher to return.

He wasn't keen. "Vince, I actually fear for my safety with those guys there," he said. I told him that if he agreed to come, I'd stay by his side during his lecture and for every meeting he had with the faculty.

Nothing adverse happened, but then again neither Urban nor Robbins showed up for any of the gatherings to which Fisher had been invited.

Another speaker I brought in was Larry Norton from nearby Mount Sinai. Larry had been one of my stellar trainees at the NCI, and he was the top medical oncologist for breast cancer in the country. He understood the intricacies of the dosing and scheduling of anticancer drugs to get the best results. But he was encountering skepticism at Mount Sinai. The doctors there found his attention to detail and his insistence on using high doses—which were more effective—too tedious. They tried to divert patients away from him by telling them that he'd give them big doses of drugs that would make them sicker, neglecting to mention that the drugs would keep them alive.

We managed to hire Zvi Fuks, one of the best radiotherapists in the world, from Israel, completing the process my predecessor had gotten started. Zvi promptly began upgrading the run-down department of radiotherapy, purchasing $40 million worth of new equipment. Under his leadership, the department was on its way to becoming one of the best in the world.

I got rid of the questionable doctor the nurses had alerted me to and replaced him. It was only after he left that we realized how substandard his care had been. I monitored the neurological status of the one surgeon with creeping paralysis, asking his team to run a check on him before each operation (he was perfectly agreeable to it), and kept a close eye on the other drinker. Whatever his habits outside the hospital, he was a great surgeon and continued to be one.

We brought in someone new to run the leukemia program. And I managed to get Larry Norton in to run our breast cancer department.

It was Evelyn Lauder, wife of Leonard Lauder, son of the cosmetics industry giant Estée Lauder, who opened the purse for clinical care. Evelyn had first consulted with me for a breast cancer diagnosis. She was under the care of a popular breast doctor at a nearby institution. But what she needed was Larry Norton's new approach to chemotherapy, and I said so. So she wanted to transfer her care to me and MSKCC.

Larry had just arrived, so I decided to transfer her to his care. I knew my boss would care about the new VIP coming to the hospital. It was a Friday afternoon, and she was scheduled to see Larry on Monday morning.

Marks panicked. We had not yet found a good place for Larry. His office was in a dilapidated room with a dumbwaiter chute. "No way Evelyn Lauder can be allowed to see that," he said.

I shrugged. I'd come from the NCI, where everything was a shade of government green. "She's more interested in the new treatment we're going to offer her," I said. "She knows Larry just got here. Don't worry."

Apparently, he didn't heed my advice. Instead, he called in MSKCC's architect on Friday evening and ordered that Norton's office be converted into a new suite by Monday. No expense was spared. It was gorgeous.

Despite Marks's Herculean effort, Lauder ended up seeing our poor outpatient facilities. Shocked, she spearheaded a drive to raise the money for a new $25 million outpatient breast center, making generous contributions herself.

Buoyed by this success, I persuaded Marks and the board to use the better part of $50 million, gained from the sale of the patent MSKCC owned on a new biologic drug, for more outpatient programs. As a result, MSKCC was on its way to becoming a leader in convenient, well-kept outpatient facilities.

But I was now constantly clashing with Marks. He was an excellent administrator and a good laboratory worker but had no sense for the clinic. He thought I was after his job. I thought he was overly concerned with growing the center's already significant endowment rather than building clinical programs.

Our weekly meetings in his office became increasingly contentious as we fought over where to allocate resources. I frequently found myself stomping my foot on the rug in his twentieth-floor office on top of the hospital, pointing down to where hundreds of patients were in the process of receiving care. "Are we running a bank or a hospital?" I'd shout.

Finally, after five years, Marks told me that he wanted me to resign if I couldn't change my ways. The truth was, as a former director of the NCI, I was too used to being in control. Realistically, I couldn't change, and I didn't really want to work there if I had to. I agreed to step down.

Marks called a meeting of the department chairs to announce my departure. I wasn't there, but one of my former colleagues was. Later, he told me that Marks had said, "The problem with Vince is that he wants to cure cancer."

The person who relayed this to me said that he and the other chairs were quite astonished by the remark. I thought it was actually a nice compliment.

The staff asked me to give a final grand round before I left. I gave it to a packed crowd in the same lecture hall where I'd been castigated for MOPP years before. I gave my vision of where the field was going and how that should affect MSKCC. Marks was standing in the back of the auditorium. When I finished, the applause began and grew. Everyone stood and kept applauding. They wouldn't stop. I finally had to walk out of the auditorium. Coming to MSKCC had been the right call, and so had doing what I'd done, even though it had cost me a job.

I passed Marks on my way out and smiled and nodded my head. He didn't look very happy, but I was.

Meanwhile, I got a call from Gerry Burrow. He'd been trying to recruit me to the University of California for years, but I hadn't wanted to move to the West Coast. Now he called and said he'd just become dean of the Yale School of Medicine and wanted to know if I'd take the job as director of Yale Cancer Center. I took it.

Going to Yale would bring my career full circle in some ways. I'd trained there decades earlier. The dean had been chief resident during my Yale residency, so I knew him well and liked him. Plus, going to one of the university-based centers would complete my tour of the system through which cancer care was delivered.

As I have mentioned, the National Cancer Act had called for fifteen centers to be built with the original funding, with the goal of a center in each state, ultimately. But how to get them set up, and quickly, had been a challenge. I was chief of medicine at the NCI when the National Cancer Act was passed and senior enough to sit in on the NCAB meetings at which the board discussed what to do about building new centers. Though it was protocol for the director of the NCI to lead these meetings, Carl Baker had turned them over to Benno Schmidt, who was also the chair of the newly created three-person President's Cancer Panel.

The question was, should we build new freestanding cancer centers, modeled after the existing ones, like Sloan Kettering? Or, to speed things along, should we create cancer centers within university medical centers, where the buildings and beds already existed and many research dollars were already invested?

The NCI's new budget was generous for that day, but only $200 million had been authorized for construction of research facilities over five years. That wasn't enough to cover construction of fifteen new freestanding centers, even then. Plus, if it was all spent on building cancer centers, there would be none left to build new laboratories. The numbers indicated we should go for university-based cancer centers.

Despite this, Benno had favored freestanding cancer centers. So had Mary Lasker, another NCAB member. Mary had a profound mistrust of academia. She thought it was only interested in basic research and disdained anything having to do with clinical research or the clinical applications of research. She worried that universities might take the money and toss it all toward basic research, leaving patients high and dry.

But most of the other NCAB members were affiliated with university medical centers, so the sentiment went their way. The issue was not an easy one, and discussions about how to create the centers continued over the course of 1972. Eventually, the vote went in favor of the university center model, which would create matrix centers—centers that were embedded within the existing space and resources from the universities, using the hospitals for patients and research labs from the medical school, and borrowing staff from both, to care for patients and do the research.

It was one of the only times I'd seen Mary Lasker and Benno Schmidt on the same side of a losing debate. As a fallback position, Mary tried to impose guidelines for center eligibility. But she was overruled, once again, by the university people.

The truth was that the universities hadn't particularly welcomed the war on cancer and didn't like the concept of the cancer centers, either. Mary had been right to be mistrustful. The focus, for them, was exclusively on basic science—science that happened in the lab and was performed not with a patient in mind but rather to get at some elusive truth.

Academia thought a program that mandated a clinical program would divert money away from research. The schools coveted the money the NCI provided, but many of them had little interest in cancer, especially if it required coordinated, targeted research that was meant to have direct application to patients.

When I became director of the NCI's Division of Cancer Treatment in 1974, I had a great deal of interaction with the cancer centers as I tried to get them more involved in developing new treatments. As director of the NCI, my perception was that they were floundering.

In fact, Yale had recruited me from Memorial Sloan Kettering as director in an attempt to save its center. It was in danger of losing its status as an NCI-designated comprehensive cancer center—for the second time—because it had repeatedly failed to live up to expectations. Its grant was due for renewal, and it had little to show that it deserved the money.

Yale was strong on basic science but not great on the clinical front—despite having been the birthplace of chemotherapy. Every major advance in the clinic in the treatment of breast and colorectal cancers and the leukemias and lymphomas had occurred with little or no participation by doctors at Yale Cancer Center. I thought the place had promise if it could build up the clinical side of the center. It didn't even have a center—a physical building—devoted to cancer patients. But Burrow had promised me full authority and his support for a new cancer building.

After being director of the NCI for eight years, and taking on Sloan Kettering, I thought, how bad could it be? The answer: pretty bad.

A special grant system was set up at the NIH to handle the NCI Cancer Centers Program. The applications for the grants, called CCSGs (Cancer Center Support Grants), or core grants for short, are monstrous tomes, each more than a thousand pages long. They usually take a center director a year to assemble and are viewed by the school as the main reason why they have a center director. Putting the grant application together occupies way too much of the time of a director whose efforts should be focused on advancing cancer management and research. These grants are not very large, either, and do not provide money to support clinical faculty or the research they do. Half of the core grants' money goes to supporting shared laboratory resources.

Most of these grants are awarded for a period of five years. And an institution cannot just decide to submit a center grant for review; it has to first get the NCI's permission even to be considered.

A major consideration is the amount of grant money the university medical center has already received. If the NCI agrees to accept a center grant, and a grant is submitted for review, a team of twenty or so physicians and scientists, most of whom work at or are directors of other NCI centers—in other words, in competition for the same dollars—are selected by the NCI to visit the institution to review the programs outlined in the grant and score them.

This is referred to as the site visit. When the reviewers visit, they evaluate the institutional commitment to the cancer center, taking into account such things as space and money, and they pay special attention to the required authorities of the director and to the success of research programs in meeting predefined benchmarks. These range from publication in scientific journals, to evidence of program meetings, productive use of shared resources, and the extent of collaboration among center members.

The grant application, which normally takes a year to produce, was due the day I was to arrive, July 1, 1993. My predecessor, unhappy about not being reappointed, had done nothing to prepare it. I went to the NCI with Burrow and asked for a three-month extension, which was granted.

I then took the month of July to get to know my way around. In August, I began to solicit help from the center's program directors to prepare the application. But being that it was August—vacation time in academia—most were gone. I did what I could and then instituted a crash effort in September. We just met the submission deadline of October 1, 1993.

While I knew Yale was a halfhearted cancer center, I was stunned by what I'd found. Twenty years after it had received cancer center designation from the NCI, nothing was going on. The focused research programs required by the NCI were a joke. Yale's clinical trials program barely existed and was housed in a closet.

In 1980, Yale had received $1.2 million in construction money from the NCI, which it had used to build new laboratories. Meanwhile, the clinical facilities were run-down, cramped, and scattered all over the place. Radiation therapy was located in a building two blocks away from the medical oncology clinics, where people received chemotherapy. Quick and easy consultation was not possible.

The general surgical clinics were a few floors above the medical oncology clinic, but if a patient was to have a breast biopsy, a needle would be inserted when the patient was in the clinic and then, clad in a hospital gown, she would be trundled by wheelchair almost three blocks to another building where the biopsy took place. None of the other surgical or diagnostic specialties were nearby.

The facilities were all located in the departments where they originated. There was no central location for the cancer facility; there wasn't even a sign anywhere indicating there *was* a cancer center at Yale. Inevitably, patient care suffered in this system.

The problem at Yale was the same problem at most university-based centers: the medical school and the hospital had different missions. The medical school saw its mission as teaching and research, the search for new knowledge. It was there to turn out the doctors of tomorrow. But the hospital's main focus was on staying in the black. A good program to a hospital is one that attracts patients and brings in income.

The missions of medical schools and their hospitals rarely overlap. In most cases, hospitals are separate organizations. On top of that, targeted programs like those called for by the National Cancer Act were anathema to medical schools. The mantra of these centers is "investigator-initiated research." This is visualized as research ideas coming straight from an investigator's mind unencumbered by any outside influence. In other words, the R01 grant.

And cancer centers are supposed to support and develop doctors who can both do research and apply the results of research. The buzzword for this is "translational research"—research that facilitates the transfer of an important lab discovery to the clinic.

But the tenure system at universities doesn't support that. And the goal, for most doctors at universities, is to become a tenured professor. And you cannot get tenured if you don't have R01 grants. That's because medical schools at major universities rely on this grant money to support the salaries of their doctors and scientists and to meet overhead. People who work in labs are those who get R01 grants. Those who do clinical research—on people, generally—do not. Or they don't get enough. And they can't get promoted without them.

In a tenure system, in most cases, you have ten years to make professor, during which time you are expected to publish, and publish a lot. If you don't make tenure, you are required to leave, and the whole world will know that you didn't pass muster. And ten papers will not get you promoted. Rarely will twenty do it. Usually, you need to publish a minimum of fifty papers in prestigious journals to be considered for promotion to professor with tenure. People who work in laboratories who can churn out experiments in weeks can do this, even if they don't make major discoveries. (And most don't.)

If you're lucky enough to have a good idea for a study involving human subjects, and you can find funds to support it, if it requires a clinical trial, you're cooked. Because it'll probably take you a year to set it up, three years to gather enough patients, and five years of follow-up. That's nine years. Even if it is a brilliant idea, you may get one or two papers out of it at most before your time is up. There are no second chances.

As a consequence, the very best clinical investigators, the ones who change paradigms in their fields, are usually encouraged to leave unless another way can be found to promote them outside the tenure system. Hence what you often see in university-based cancer centers is a fast turnover of talented clinicians, and patients wondering why the doctor who began their care is now gone.

At freestanding centers such as MSKCC, you are knee-deep in doctors for every type of cancer, but, as I have mentioned, the risk is that they might have gotten entrenched in a certain way of approaching the disease. At university centers like Yale, there were often too few doctors and not enough expertise in each specialty. Because doctors didn't necessarily stay for long, the strengths of the centers, like all centers created by the National Cancer Act, varied from year to year.

I discovered, too, that the budget of a cancer center was something of a pretense. A center such as Yale may have $75 million of NCI money attributed to it, but only $2 million would be in the form of the core grant managed by the center's director. Most of the rest came in the form of R01 grants, which had been applied for independently by investigators at the medical school and distributed around various departments. None of this money, the investigators involved, or the space used was really under the authority of the center's director.

So university cancer centers had borrowed staff, almost no authority, a patchwork budget, and in many cases facilities scattered all over hell and gone. The construction money for cancer centers largely went elsewhere.

Yale had been an NCI-designated cancer center for more than twenty years at a cost to the NCI of more than $40 million in the core grant (that is, not including money that came in via R01 grants), and it had yet to get its act together.

When I saw the state of affairs at Yale, I complained to the center's associate director, a brilliant cell biologist. He actually bragged that he had never had a meeting of his own research program—a program that was supposed to unify the research efforts at Yale Cancer Center—in the preceding five years.

When I expressed concern to another scientist regarding our ability to get the grant renewed, this distinguished immunologist and head of the center's immunology research program was dismissive. "Come on, Vince, no way NCI is going to reject a grant from its prior director," he said. I wasn't so sure.

Before I'd left the NCI, I'd asked the National Cancer Advisory Board to develop stricter guidelines for centers in order to continue as NCI-designated cancer centers. It had taken six years, but the board had done it. There were seven standards to be met. The most important was institutional commitment, measured in resources supplied to the center. Then there were demonstrated authorities of the director over space, personnel, and research dollars. The new guidelines also called for a viable clinical trials program and evidence of functioning, organized research programs; a significant amount of research dollars in place; and a broad enough array of research programs, including those on prevention, to qualify as a comprehensive center.

Ironically, Yale was going to be in the first group to be reviewed under the new guidelines. I knew there was no way we could meet them.

When the site visit team arrived four months later, it was an uneasy time for me. We played the game. We stretched the truth and told them that hallway conversations were formal program meetings, and the dean assured them that I was truly in charge. The president of the hospital promised continued unyielding support, which he never gave. Even the new president of Yale, Rick Levin, promised the site visit team that the school would have a new center building by the time of the next grant review in five years.

In the executive session where the site visit team meets with the center director alone, I mumbled that it had been difficult to meet the new guidelines that I had set in motion. One member of the site visit team, a former trainee of mine and now a center director himself, said in a stage whisper, "Poetic justice."

The site visitors told me they were disappointed in Yale's institutional commitment to the center, disappointed in the stunted section of medical oncology, and horrified by the lack of clinical studies. But they were reassured that with my leadership things would change.

We really should not have been funded, but we were. The distinguished immunologist had been right: it was hard to reject the grant of a former NCI director. Yale had made the correct call in hiring me.

Though it was unusual for the former director of the NCI to be in the hot seat, it wasn't unusual for a cancer center to be funded even though it didn't deserve to be. Two cancer centers in their early days were funded despite not receiving approvable scores: the Dana-Farber Cancer Institute, in Boston, and the Fred Hutchinson Cancer Research Center, in Seattle. (Those centers actually went on to become outstanding.) In both cases, senators had intervened on their behalf and told the NCI, in no uncertain terms, that it had to fund them. But even without government intervention, the NCI has leeway in extending center grants under special circumstances, to allow a center to try to get its act together. Many centers, including Yale, Herbert Irving at Columbia, NYU, and the Sylvester Comprehensive Cancer Center at the University of Miami, have had their grants extended via political favor to avoid the embarrassment of losing NCI designation. Nonetheless, these centers also went on to be outstanding.

Twice, I got Yale's core grant approved by finessing the truth. After each round, I tried to build the center up—and tried to literally get a cancer center built. It was maddening.

The hospital and the medical school could agree on nothing. The hospital wanted no part of research programs in a center, and the medical school wanted no part of a center totally devoted to clinical cancer; the school wanted lab space. At one point, the hospital came up with its own plan to devote $25 million to a clinical facility devoted to cancer. But the dean of the medical school walked out of the meeting when he found out that it would not be building any laboratories. They even argued over names. Yale preferred Yale Cancer Center, which was, after all, what we were supposed to be. The hospital's president wanted Yale–New Haven Cancer Center. The medical school faculty rejected this because they said it made it seem as if there were no research programs associated with the center.

It all reflected a pervasive but silly business. The hospital thinks the medical school academics are snobby and pay no attention to business, and it wants the hospital brand name to be dominant. The medical school wants the hospital to recognize that the latter belongs to Yale and that the Yale name trumps all. It also doesn't want to give the impression that it works for the hospital, and it wants the hospital to use revenues to support research, which the hospital refuses to do. In fact, the hospital's charter forbids it to support research. This atmosphere had prevailed when I was a resident, and I was amazed, when I came back, to discover that nothing had changed.

At one point, the school and the hospital spent $150,000 on a consulting firm, which promptly hired one of my former staffers at the NCI, to prepare an analysis. A year later, she made a scathing presentation, recommending everything that I had suggested, including making the cancer center a joint program of the school and the hospital and supporting the recommendation for a new cancer building. This presentation took place in a small room with only a few people in attendance. The president of the hospital didn't bother to show up.

I tell you this story not to pillory Yale particularly, though it behaved badly with regard to its obligations to the war on cancer and to its patients, just as Mary Lasker had feared. The cancer centers at NYU, Columbia, Albert Einstein, Jefferson Medical College, University of

Chicago, University of California, San Diego, UCLA, University of Miami, University of Colorado, Georgetown University, Duke, University of Alabama, University of Virginia, Wake Forest University, Emory, University of Hawaii, and Northwestern University, just to name a few more typical of the genre, had virtually the same problems.

The bottom line is that despite the dream of state-of-the-art care for all people at all institutions, no one institution is right for every cancer patient. I am not saying anything new here; this is an open secret. All center directors at universities know that the NCI's cancer centers were shoehorned into an inhospitable system and that the situation needs fixing. All would like to see that change. But while they will talk about it privately, they can't say so publicly, because they may lose their grant money and their jobs. Many are even afraid to complain much at their own institutions for fear of being branded "not collegial."

I am asked to consult on some aspect of care for up to two hundred patients a year. More often than not, I refer them to doctors at well-known cancer centers, which, despite their flaws, are still where the new therapies are being developed. But my advice varies depending on the patients and the type of cancer they have. The center and doctors I refer them to often may not be at my own center, even if the patients are in the neighborhood. And it may not be the one nearest to them, either.

Centers are not one-stop shopping, as they were envisioned. Most can generally be relied on to deliver current, state-of-the-art care equivalent to the care received at any other major hospital. The United States is unique in this way. But the high-quality programs at cancer centers, the ones that lead the way in developing innovative care for cancer patients—and to which some patients need access in order to survive—are constantly in flux. In the 1970s and 1980s, the NCI, Stanford, and the Dana-Farber Cancer Center were the go-to places for lymphomas. They invented most of the treatments in use today. Stanford and the Farber are still among the best places in the country for treatment of lymphomas, but the NCI program has fallen by the wayside. The NCI, however, is now the go-to place for the treatment of metastatic melanoma and innovative approaches to immunotheraphy.

Sloan Kettering's lymphoma program was not up to the standards of a leading cancer center when I got there in the late 1980s, and it's still catching up, but it is now one of the great centers, with world-class programs in breast, pediatric, urologic, and neurological cancers, to name just a few. Yale may be the best place to go for cutaneous T cell lymphomas but not for any other type. Yale's urologic oncology program had been in abeyance for decades because, until recently, it lacked clinical investigators in medical and radiation oncology to support its excellent surgeons.

The Mayo Clinic is good for state-of-the-art care for common tumors, but I wouldn't send someone there who needed something creative or inventive. NYU's Perlmutter Cancer Center has always been a very good place for surgery for brain tumors (better, until recently, than its close neighbor Sloan Kettering) but not much else.

The best place for adult leukemia therapy is MD Anderson in Houston, Texas.

Dana-Farber has, by far, the best program for the treatment of myeloma, a bone marrow cancer. And the leadership in breast cancer, until Larry Norton came to MSKCC, has come from the cancer center at the University of Pittsburgh.

And so it goes. For every type of cancer, at every important cancer center. And these things are constantly changing.

Centers don't especially want patients to know about their deficiencies. In fact, what I've written above will make me very unpopular among many of my colleagues at cancer centers. To give you some idea of the sensitivity of the issue, let me recount an experience, from a long time ago, when treatment for Hodgkin's disease had just become established and was being offered at a handful of centers. I was on a panel with half a dozen of the country's experts on Hodgkin's. We had just described, to an audience of science writers, what an institution needed to be able to treat patients right. One reporter raised her hand and addressed a question to the chair of the panel, Dr. Saul

Rosenberg, a prominent lymphoma specialist from Stanford University. "Dr. Rosenberg, how many places in the country are capable of doing this the way you describe?" she said.

Saul looked up at the ceiling and hesitated a bit. He rubbed his chin thoughtfully. "About a dozen," he said. You could feel the next question coming before he'd finished his sentence. Indeed, every hand in the audience had shot up. "Which dozen?" said the first person called upon, asking the question they all wanted to know the answer to.

Saul was blindsided. To answer was to reveal the many institutions that did not have the capacity to treat Hodgkin's correctly. In truth, we all should have anticipated this question and should have known how to answer it tactfully. But we hadn't.

Now Saul stood in front of a microphone, the appointed responder with sixty science journalists, all of whom knew a hedge when they heard one, waiting impatiently for an answer.

In the end, Saul refused to name the dozen. But that wasn't the end of it. When the panel broke up, each of us was cornered by members of the press representing papers from different cities, wanting to know whether their center was one of the twelve.

Joann Rodgers, a diminutive but tough science writer for Baltimore's *News American*, tagged me. "Okay, Vince," she said. "Is Johns Hopkins one of those places?"

I stood paralyzed for a second, knowing the hell I faced if I answered correctly. But I answered. For one, patients had a right to know. For another, I knew that Joann, who stands all of five feet tall, was tough. She wasn't going anywhere until I answered. "No," I said, weakly.

The next day, a piece authored by Joann appeared in the *News American*, proclaiming Hopkins's failures. My phone didn't stop ringing for days. Its radiotherapist called and chewed me out, as did its medical oncologist, both of whom were good friends of mine. I had to explain to them the difference between delivering what was formerly state-of-the-art treatment, each specialty going it alone, and what the new approach was, using new treatments with all specialties collaborating at the outset.

What I had said was true. At that time, your best chance of being cured of Hodgkin's disease was to go to one of about a dozen places in the United States. Johns Hopkins wasn't one of them. The truth hurts. And it also hurts referrals.

The bald truth is that the NCI university cancer center model is broken.* And if you are diagnosed with a cancer that might be fatal, you cannot assume that the nearest cancer center has the necessary expertise for your particular cancer.

There's no question that cancer centers are key to the control of cancer in this country. But all centers are not alike, and no center is all things to all people. Centers are about the people who staff them. The very best go-to places are those where they're provided with the resources to practice as a team, in an environment that offers the freedom to exercise their talents on behalf of the patient.

But getting to these places, and these doctors, requires inside knowledge that most patients don't have. That's why I am so often guiding friends and friends of friends to different centers. And that's why PDQ (Physician Data Query) is so helpful. Going to centers that aren't near you also requires flexible insurance companies, which some people don't have. And the Affordable Care Act (ACA) promises to make this worse. The focus of the ACA is cost control, and the mechanism to monitor this is the Independent Payment Advisory Board, which mimics the British National Institute for Health and Care Excellence (NICE), which determines if new treatments are cost-effective before allowing payment. NICE, or Not So Nice, as I have called it, regularly determines that new lifesaving cancer therapies are not cost-effective, essentially rationing cancer care. In any system of rationing care, new approaches to cancer treatment are always

---

*Gordon Zubrod and Tom Frei, two of the people instrumental in creating a fertile environment for discovery and progress at the NCI, eventually left the NCI to try to work within university programs. Zubrod found a disorganized cancer center at the University of Miami and was unable to fix it before he retired. Frei went to Harvard. When I complained to him once about the state of affairs at Yale, he said, "Vince, the first five years at Harvard were the worst five years of my life."

at the bottom of the list. And because the field is changing so rapidly, much of tomorrow's care is being invented today. New therapies are likely to go uncovered, making them inaccessible to patients.

There are incredibly promising therapies out there. If used to their fullest potential for all patients, I believe we could cure an additional 100,000 patients a year.

But this requires teams, and teamwork requires facilities and other resources devoted to clinical cancer and judgment calls by experienced physicians.

The problems are fixable. Sloan Kettering is just one example. Yale is another.

After I left Sloan Kettering, I kept a copy of the strategic plan I'd made for the institution in my desk. Amazingly, after I left, it began to implement the plan. Over the course of several years, I'd hear from friends still at MSKCC that another piece of the plan had just been put in place. One day, after receiving such a call, I crossed the last item off the list. In the end, it had done them all. MSKCC is now living up to its potential.

And now so is Yale.

In 2006, thirty-two years after receiving its NCI designation, we broke ground on the Yale Cancer Center building. Finally, Yale would have a cancer center with an actual "center." But, ironically, when the building was dedicated, it was called the Smilow Cancer Hospital, after the major donor. Nowhere on the building is there mention of Yale Cancer Center. Yet for the first time in its long history, Yale is harnessing its research programs in the interest of cancer patients.

Yale has matured, as have many other centers, in the past ten years. But many were useless for the first fifteen years of their existence. As a clinician, or a family member, you have to wonder how many people we have lost to what you might charitably call the growing pains of easing into the mandates called for in the war on cancer.

Despite all that I have told you, the United States has the best cancer care in the world. Not all patients receive their care at cancer centers, nor do they need to. Much of cancer care can be delivered at community hospitals. It's the critical cases—those with a less than 15 percent survival rate or diagnosed at a late stage—that most rely on what is supposed to be the cutting edge. The state of the art in cancer management is changing on a daily basis, and state-of-the-art treatments are developed at cancer centers. So for someone who has a serious cancer that threatens his or her life, it is often advantageous to go to a cancer center where a new therapy is being developed.

But, as a clinician, if someone put me on the spot, as Joann Rodgers once did, and asked me if the cancer centers have always done the best by their patients, I would have to answer: we could have done better.

10

THE DEATH OF CANCER

Since the launching of the war on cancer in 1971, we have spent more than $100 billion on cancer research. You might well ask, what do we have to show for it?

Not much, if you believe what you read in the press. "Rethinking the War on Cancer," wrote Sharon Begley in *Newsweek* on September 5, 2008.[1] "Forty Years' War: Advances Elusive in the Drive to Cure Cancer," wrote Gina Kolata on the front page of *The New York Times* on April 23, 2009.[2] And in 2013, the journalist Clifton Leaf published a book called *The Truth in Small Doses: Why We're Losing the War on Cancer—and How to Win It*, an outgrowth of a 2004 article he had written for *Fortune* magazine.[3]

It has become a drumbeat in the media: we're losing the war on cancer.

These articles, and others like them, are wrong. We have learned an enormous amount about cancer since the war on cancer was launched, and we're learning more all the time. The evidence is clear: we *are* winning the war on cancer.

For one thing, mortality statistics have completely turned around. Overall mortality, despite predictions to the contrary, began to decline in 1990 and has dropped 25 percent since then. And mortality for common cancers has dropped as well: for breast cancer, 25 percent; for colon cancer, 45 percent; for prostate cancer, 68 percent; and for leukemias and lymphomas even more.

This has huge consequences not only for people's lives but for the American economy. An independent analysis by the economists Kevin Murphy and Robert Topel at the University of Chicago looked at the economic benefit of improvements in the health of the workforce.[4] The biggest return on investment in health came from cardiovascular diseases, where mortality decreases already seen can account for an approximately $30 trillion return to the economy. But they found that for every 20 percent drop in cancer mortality, about $10 trillion is added to the economy. So the overall 25 percent mortality decline so far is worth more than a thousand times what has been invested in cancer research. On an economic basis alone, the war on cancer has been a great investment.

Not only are cures happening more often, but in the cases in which they're not, cancer has become, for many people, a chronic, manageable disease—not a killer. And the startling thing is that most of the mortality declines are due to refinement and more widespread use of old technology: mutilating surgeries, such as the radical mastectomy, have given way to more refined ones that still got the job done; radiotherapy equipment has become more refined, allowing radiotherapy to be delivered to the tumor without killing the normal tissue surrounding it; drugs have been developed to prevent nausea and vomiting, the bane of the existence of chemotherapists, so people can tolerate drug treatment. All of this has made it possible to use old treatments better, not only by themselves, but together. Survival has improved, and patients feel better about treatment. Meanwhile, basic research paid for by the war on cancer has taught us so much that as it works its way into the clinic, the best of the war on cancer is yet to come. The press should be celebrating the victory, not moaning about the loss.

Part of the reason for this progress is the paradigm shifts that have occurred in our thinking about cancer.

There have been three such shifts in cancer treatment in the past fifty years. The first was the recognition that combination chemotherapy could cure advanced cancer. That led to the decline in mortality of the leukemias and the lymphomas in which the original work was done. And it gave birth to the use of adjuvant chemotherapy—cancer drugs paired with surgery and/or radiotherapy—that led to the decline in mortality of common cancers like those of the breast and the colon.

The second paradigm shift was the result of research that gave us proof of principle that targeted therapy—drugs aimed at specific molecular lesions that characterize certain cancers—was successful and that it could convert a previously fatal leukemia into a chronic disease that did not reduce the patient's life span. This finding is now being applied to common tumors such as lung cancer and melanoma.

The third paradigm shift was the understanding that immunotherapy—turning the patients' immune defenses against cancer—can work in a majority of patients. Though recent, this finding has already had a major impact on patients with advanced melanoma, formerly a tumor highly resistant to treatment, and very advanced leukemias and lymphomas.

All of these shifts have not only helped to cure cancer and to extend lives but also changed the experience of having cancer. For many patients, brutal treatments such as disfiguring amputations are a thing of the past. Culturally, everything has changed.

People diagnosed with cancer no longer have to go into hiding or risk pariah status. Cancer is a disease that's out in the open, so much so that people wear the colors of the cause. Every October, pink coffee lids, pink ribbons, pink shoes on football players, and pink baseball bats emerge, symbols of breast cancer awareness. People who have cancer are now seen as warriors—people who are fighting back and, what's more, people with a shot at winning—not victims.

As to what we've learned, it's breathtaking. I'm going to explain the progress in two stages. First, I'll describe what we've learned about cancer. This is a devil we know far, far better than we did when the war on cancer began. Second, I'll talk about the treatments that have come from the war on cancer and how they are changing cancer for many people into a chronic disease—not a killer.

In March 2011, I picked up a copy of *Cell*, a leading scientific journal, and noticed an article titled "Hallmarks of Cancer: The Next Generation."[5] It stopped me cold. For one thing, one of the authors was Bob Weinberg. Anything with Weinberg's name on it gets my attention. A founding member of the Whitehead Institute for Biomedical Research and a professor of biology at MIT, Weinberg did some of the original work showing that specific genes, called oncogenes, could cause cancer in rodents. This laid the foundation for our fundamental molecular understanding of the disease.

Not only is Bob a brilliant scientist, but he also happens to be a really good writer. One of his efforts is *The Biology of Cancer*, a textbook that I find so compelling I keep a copy on the reading stand of my stationary bike and read a bit of it every day.[6] It's that good.

The Weinberg paper on the hallmarks of cancer was not just any paper. Eleven years earlier, Bob and his co-author, Douglas Hanahan, Ph.D., published an article in the same journal called "The Hallmarks of Cancer," in which they wrote about six traits that all cancer cells have in common.[7]

The new study updated and extended the work in the earlier study. It painted a big picture: If all kinds of cancers share six important traits, then that dramatically shrinks the number of targets we have to attack to fight cancer. Go after those six traits, and we can have effects on many kinds of cancers.

The two papers have collectively been cited in other research papers more than fifteen thousand times. Most authors do not get that many citations for all of their papers combined in their entire career. The first paper is, to date, the most cited paper in the history of *Cell*, meaning countless other scientists refer to this paper when writing their own. It's *that* critical to the current thinking on cancer.

In the second paper, published in 2011, Weinberg and Hanahan had refined their descriptions of the original hallmarks using information gleaned from animal studies and biochemical assays, or measurements, that didn't exist a decade ago. And they added two new ones. I knew when I picked it up it was going to be a riveting paper, and it was.

The hallmarks of all cancer cells, per Weinberg and Hanahan's paper, are the following: sustained proliferative signaling; evasion of growth suppressors; resistance to cell death; avoidance of immune destruction; the ability to induce angiogenesis; the deregulation of cellular energetics; the ability to enable replicative immortality; and the activation of invasion and metastases.

Now let me translate.

A cancer cell starts as a perfectly normal adult cell packed tightly, shoulder to shoulder, with other similar cells. They can talk to each other by communicating through their contact points, like pressing a buzzer on an intercom. Depending on which organ the cells are in, the signals generally say, *Sit still, do your job, make proteins, excrete waste, but, as much as you might like to, don't even think about dividing.*

But, unbeknownst to the soon-to-be cancer cell, some changes have been taking place behind the scenes. The cell genes that suppress unwanted, dangerous growth might have been altered by a mutation or by inheriting defective genes in a way that makes them unable to respond. These cells aren't cancerous yet, but they are primed to become cancer cells.

These abnormalities can be inherited, as with some familial cancer syndromes, usually apparent from a careful family history. Or the abnormalities can occur because our genes are bombarded with materials that damage them (for example, chemicals in cigarette smoke that cause lung cancer) and bring about structural changes known as mutations (as occur in colon cancer). Or a cancer-causing virus captures the genes that control growth to allow the cell to replicate (as the papilloma virus does to cause cervical cancer). That's okay, as long as the genes responsible for growth behave themselves.

It takes another incident—another mutation, or extra copies of the gene, or an abnormality in the controlling element of the gene—to cause cancer. The cell receives a steady signal to grow and begins to divide. It continues, with one eye looking back over its shoulder, fully expecting a rap on the head from the suppressor gene for disobeying orders. But if that suppressor is broken, the rap on the head doesn't come.

These are the first two hallmarks of cancer: sustained willy-nilly growth; and a deactivation of the braking system present in normal cells. Then the cancer cell is like a car rolling down a hill—all acceleration and no brakes.

The life of a budding cancer cell is not that easy; this is why we don't all die of cancer as children. Many cells primed to become cancer do not progress to that stage. The would-be cancer cell must face other immediate challenges if it is going to continue its course. Evading the cell's suicide mechanism is one.

When we develop as embryos, we go through stages that mimic our distant ancestors. We develop gills for a time, for instance, and webbed fingers and toes. We don't have them at birth, because Mother Nature put a cell-suicide system in place which signals cells that are not wanted to commit suicide. And the mechanism stays in place as we grow into adulthood, when it's used to tell cells that have incurred dangerous cell damage to commit suicide. So it's hardly surprising that from a cancer cell's perspective, this mechanism is one of the first controls that has to go. With suppressors inactivated, cells that have incurred damage can no longer be forced to commit suicide.

Next there is the immune system designed to recognize and destroy anything foreign and dangerous to the host. The immune system can ferret out rogue cells and send an army of assassin lymphocytes to kill them. This immune reaction can be dangerous in adults if the immune system goes after the wrong cells. So normal cells have a system to deactivate a harmful immune reaction. When this deactivation fails, we develop autoimmune diseases like lupus and inflammatory arthritis. The budding cancer cell co-opts this system, inactivates it, and fools the immune system into ignoring it.

These are the first four hallmarks of cancer cells: growth, deactivation of the braking system, the loss of the suicide mechanism, and the trickery with the immune system. They may not emerge exactly in that order, and what I've described may take place slowly, over months to years, but they are the essential elements that convert a normal cell to a cancer.

But like Patton's Third Army, the cancer cell moves so fast that it runs out of fuel quickly if its supply line is not maintained. It needs a blood supply. So it co-opts the normal cells' ability to form blood vessels, an ability normally only used by adult cells to help heal wounds.

That blood can supply the nutrients the cancer cell needs. But the tumor also needs a source of building blocks for DNA synthesis. To get them, it reaches back into the bag of tricks normally only available to a developing embryo and activates a form of energy metabolism referred to as aerobic glycolysis.

Humans derive their energy from two forms of metabolism, oxidative phosphorylation and glycolysis. Oxidative phosphorylation is the preferred form and takes place in the presence of oxygen carried by the red blood cells in the bloodstream (that's what "oxidative" means). It results in the complete metabolism of nutrients to glucose and from glucose to water and carbon dioxide, which are easily excreted by the lungs and kidneys. Normal cells use it predominantly, because it's the most efficient way to generate energy, and without energy generation we would die.

Glycolysis, on the other hand, is used in normal tissue only when oxygen is in short supply—in the muscles of long-distance runners, for example—because it results in the incomplete burning of glucose. Energy-wise, it is inefficient. In the absence of oxygen, it's called anaerobic (meaning "in the absence of air") glycolysis. When it occurs in the presence of oxygen, it is highly unusual. But cancer cells prefer this method, as inefficient as it is, because the incomplete burning of glucose leaves parts of molecules behind that can be used to synthesize DNA and other large molecules that rapidly dividing cells need.

The cancer cell, like the embryo, retains the ability to switch back and forth between the two forms of metabolism, with some cells doing one and others doing the other, depending on a cell's needs at the time. This provides a big advantage over normal cells. If food is in short supply, the products of glycolysis from some cancer cells can be used to feed the cells nearby using oxidative phosphorylation, while the latter provide energy for the other cells. The cancer cell still faces the ultimate problem, however. If it and its progeny are to survive, it needs to be immortal.

As cells divide, they gradually shorten the ends of the chromosomes, called telomeres. And when the protective ends are gone, the DNA becomes sticky, and the ends of one chromosome can stick randomly to a different chromosome. When cells with stuck chromosomes try to divide, they get pulled in the wrong direction, resulting in an imbalance of chromosomes, chaotic cell division, and, most often, cell death. This is another mechanism the body uses to prevent dangerous unlimited growth. We just run out of telomeres. But the cancer cell reaches, once more, into the embryo's bag of tricks. Embryonic cells possess an enzyme, called telomerase, which constantly replenishes the ends of chromosomes so they never get sticky. Otherwise, it would wear out its telomeres even before an infant was fully formed, and growth would stop. Adult cells have no measurable telomerase, because once a fetus is formed, it doesn't need that kind of rapid growth anymore. Cancer cells reactivate telomerase.

So now the cancer cell has its growth switch locked in the on position, unchecked by suppressors. It is ignoring the cell-death mechanism, it is evading the immune system, and it has created its own blood supply and its own way of obtaining nutrients. Plus, it's immortal.

But there's more: the cancer must spread. Cancer patients, with few exceptions, die because cancer cells metastasize, or, as the British say, develop "secondaries"—deposits of cancer cells in vital organs elsewhere in the body. A breast cancer patient never dies because of the tumor in the breast. She dies when it metastasizes, or spreads, to bone and liver or brain. The patient dies from the expanding brain tumors or liver failure. A colon cancer patient rarely dies because of the tumor in his colon. He dies because the cancer cells have populated the liver and cause it to fail.

The budding cancer cell reactivates this ability to travel, which is another characteristic critical to the developing embryo. Embryos use this mechanism to move new cells around to form each of our different organs.

The scientific term for this program is the "epithelial to mesenchymal transition," or EMT for short. Recognition of the importance of the EMT in cancer is another major contribution of Bob Weinberg. The most common cancers derive from epithelial tissue in various organs. That tissue is normally immobile. Mesenchymal cells, on the other hand, can move and cross membrane barriers. When EMT happens, an immobile epithelial cancer cell becomes a mobile, invasive mesenchymal cell. The cancer cell probably does this in its quest to reach favorable areas to grow or to reach out to an area with more robust blood vessels than it can make with its own mechanism. This mobility of cancer cells is the reason surgery or radiotherapy works only in a small fraction of cancer patients. It's the reason removing a primary tumor after cells have metastasized doesn't work. That's why some form of systemic therapy is necessary for almost all cancers.

So instead of a hundred different cancers, each with its own pattern of growth, we have these eight hallmarks typical of all cancers. The importance of each of them varies with the type of cancer. For example, leukemias and lymphomas derive from cells that are normally mobile, so for them activating the EMT program is less important, because they normally travel in the bloodstream. But with few exceptions, for a cancer to kill its host, it needs all hallmarks.

Perhaps you've noted the word "embryo" several times in the preceding paragraphs. It is now clear that the cancer cell is recapitulating developmental biology. In plainer terms, it thinks it's a fertilized egg on its way to becoming an embryo, and it uses the powerful growth machinery of the early embryo, normally shut down in adulthood, to fire its growth and development. You can look at cancer, then, as a failure in the control of the delicate cellular machinery that evolved to prevent embryos from becoming monsters. This sounds fantastic, I know, but it's true. There are cancers that, when removed, are found to have hair and teeth and other tissues. They're called teratomas, from the Greek word *teras*—meaning monster.

I should mention something else Weinberg noted. In recent years, it has also become apparent that inflammation can increase the risk of cancer, because cancer cells, or even precancerous cells, can receive growth signals from normal cells found in inflammatory tissue. So tumor-promoting inflammation is another enabling characteristic of cancer. Evidence of the importance of inflammation has been apparent for decades. Inflammatory bowel disease is associated with a high risk of colon cancer. Gallstones and cholecystitis (inflammation of the gallbladder) are associated with an increased incidence of gallbladder cancer. Lung cancer sometimes occurs in the scars of old tubercular lesions. And Burkitt's lymphoma, in Africa, is seen almost exclusively in areas where falciparum malaria is endemic, causing inflammation.

The hallmarks of cancer, then, are acquired characteristics that cancer cells need to survive and grow. Without them, cancer cells are not a threat to life. Prevent them from developing, and a normal cell will not become a cancer cell. Get to a growing tumor mass before it fully develops all the hallmarks, and it can be cured by local means like surgery or radiotherapy. Shut these hallmarks down in a metastatic cancer, and a growing cancer is stopped in its tracks.

We are now able to do all of the above.

Most of our current successful systemic treatments have been aimed at a single one of these hallmarks. For example, chemotherapy, and most of the new targeted therapies, attack the first hallmark discussed—sustained proliferative signaling. Immunotherapy restores the surveillance function of the immune system. Weinberg's hallmarks paper introduces the prospect of another paradigm shift. Just as we learned that a combination of drugs was needed to cure lymphomas, leukemias, and breast and colorectal cancers, we now know that to be most successful in dealing with the hallmarks of cancer, we need to attack more than one.

Attacking multiple hallmarks at the same time requires that we do complex clinical trials of a new kind. We can randomly combine a variety of drugs to try to attack multiple hallmarks simultaneously, but the analysis of such studies would be a statistical nightmare. The new studies need to be planned using the wiring diagram of the cancer cell in question as the blueprint. And they must be conducted in a radically different way from conventional studies. These studies hold extraordinary promise, but they are virtually impossible under the government's current regulations. Normally, when we test a new treatment, we establish a protocol and hold that constant during the trial to isolate the effect of the treatment. But in these new multi-hallmark trials, we will need to monitor the effects and adjust the approach on the fly—during the trial—to fully use all the information at our disposal. Current regulations make it difficult to get that kind of study approved.

In 1971, when the National Cancer Act was first proposed, we knew nothing about the hallmarks of cancer, of course. We did know there were rogue cells, but we didn't know how a normal cell became cancerous or how cancer cells could overwhelm normal cells.

Back when we created MOPP we didn't know the first thing about how a cancer cell thought. Sure, we knew where it started and how it tended to spread—what we refer to as the natural history of a cancer. And we knew how it behaved untouched by human hands. But did we know how it thought? No.

As a result of the war on cancer, the cancer cell is no longer a black box; it's a blueprint. And we can read blueprints. We understand the cancer cell's stages, how it thinks, what drives it. And we have the tools to attack each of the steps on the way to malignancy. There isn't a question about cancer we can't address, at this point, without the expectation of a usable answer.

As optimistic as I am, I don't think there will ever be a world in which cancer doesn't occur. It's in our biology. In the millions of cell divisions that take place in our bodies every day, there are too many opportunities for mistakes. And some of those mistakes will activate a cancer hallmark and give rise to cancer.

We can prevent it, to some extent, by avoiding the things that make those mistakes more prone to happen, like smoking. And we can take advantage of medication that seems, in some cases, to prevent those mistakes. For instance, nonsteroidal anti-inflammatory drugs, like Aleve and Motrin and even low-dose aspirin, prevent the development of colon polyps, the precursor of colon cancers. We also have drugs that can prevent breast, prostate, and head and neck cancers. But cells will be cells. Mistakes happen and will continue to happen—giving rise to cancer. I do, however, think we're heading for a time when we'll be able to cure almost all cancers. And those that we can't cure as readily will be converted to chronic, manageable diseases.

But what do we mean when we call a disease chronic? The cold and the flu are acute illnesses. They last days or at most weeks. Chronic diseases last months or years, or for life. Diabetes, hypertension, and arthritis are chronic diseases. Once you have them, they're yours forever. But they can be controlled; you can live with them.

Cancer qualifies as a chronic disease now because each case usually plays out over several years. But while other chronic diseases just shorten life somewhat, or are disabling, they are not quickly fatal. That's the difference. Cancer is the most curable chronic disease. But it is more often fatal as well.

So when I say we want to convert most cancers into chronic diseases, I mean we want cancer patients we can't cure to more closely resemble those with diabetes or arthritis—to live out a normal or near-normal life span while managing the condition. Immortality is not our goal here, just a normal life, free from the gnawing worry that a premature death is lurking just around the corner. We can worry about immortality after we cure cancer.

But we also need to ask what we mean by "cure." Believe it or not, the definition is controversial. In fact, it varies from cancer to cancer.

For each stage of every cancer, there is a "critical period," a time period after which the likelihood of recurrence in the future is small. For breast cancer patients who are found to have tumor cells in their lymph nodes at the time of operation and who are treated with anti-cancer drugs in the post-op period, you get a good idea of their long-term prognosis by about eighteen months after first treatment. If no tumor reappears, then the chances of recurrence are small. After five years, the chance is very small. Patients with advanced Hodgkin's disease who go into a complete remission with chemotherapy and don't have a recurrence after four years of follow-up, with no further treatment, have very little chance of having to deal with another bout of the disease. I have seen this occur only a few times in my entire career. For the most aggressive form of lymphoma, the diffuse large B-cell lymphoma, the critical period is even shorter, only two years. That's because these tumors grow so fast that if you don't eradicate all of the cancer cells, they will grow back and kill you quickly. Even for a rarely cured tumor like cancer of the pancreas, if you are free of disease four years after surgery, you are cured. If you aren't, it will let you know by then. Some cancers are less predictable. Patients with surgically removed deep melanomas, for example, can recur even after having been free of disease for years.

In my opinion, when there is less than a 10 percent chance of the cancer recurring after a patient passes his or her cancer's critical period, then the person should be told that, in all likelihood, he or she is cured.

There are some oncologists—I call them DOs, or doubting oncologists—who would pale at what I have just written. That's because most oncologists are nearly phobic about using the word "cure." They hedge their bets because they don't want to be wrong or they're too pessimistic. When I talk about cancer to young doctors and use the word "cure," I can almost hear the collective intake of breath. Some brave soul may even ask, "How can you be sure they are cured?" Well, I can't be absolutely sure, which is why I say "in all likelihood." But when the data tell me the chances are nine to one that the patient will stay free of disease, I tell them I like the odds. I always emphasize the curability of the disease whenever I can. Hedging makes the doctor feel better, but the patient feels worse.

Living with cancer is not something most patients want to do. They want to live without it. When patients get past the high-risk period, they are cured. And in my mind, they also no longer have a chronic disease. The DOs are paling again. "What? Are you crazy? Once a cancer patient, always a cancer patient, right?" But let's be fair here. If you are cured of pneumonia, you are not always a pneumonia patient. You "had" pneumonia. Why should it be different with cancer? When we say we want to convert cancer into a chronic disease, we don't mean living free of cancer after a diagnosis. That's a cure. We mean keeping people alive *with their cancer* for a near-normal life span.

But no one is ever cured of a metastatic cancer that doesn't first go into complete remission. Setting the goal on getting a complete remission is so important I thought about naming this book "Complete Remission." Unfortunately, many young doctors don't understand this issue, either. A lot of cancer doctors try to settle for less when in pursuit of creating a chronic state. But they mistake a few extra months of life for a real chronic state—a long life with cancer.

One avenue some of these doctors use is long-term, low-dose chemotherapy. The literature is replete with how well tolerated this approach is: it produces much less in the way of side effects. While immunotherapy may be an exception, it's clear that low, nontoxic doses of chemotherapy are no match for cancer. Rarely do you see patients on this treatment go into complete remission. The real toxicity of low-dose chemotherapy is premature death. If your doctor recommends it, head for the nearest exit.

This doesn't mean every patient should be treated with very high doses, either. Full or higher doses of cancer drugs, used in combination, work only in tumors that are known to be sensitive to each drug individually, as was the case using both VAMP and MOPP. In tumors that are known to be insensitive to specific drugs, increasing the doses only causes more side effects. But in sensitive tumors, increasing the doses can mean the difference between cure and failure.

Frank Schabel, who worked at the Southern Research Institute in Birmingham, Alabama, with Howard Skipper, did a set of experiments that were very telling about the effect of full doses of chemotherapy on the ability to cure a metastatic tumor. He implanted mouse sarcomas into groups of mice and watched the sarcomas grow until the mice had lots of measurable tumors in their lungs. Then he treated them with combinations of cancer drugs. At full doses, all of the mice went into complete remission. That is, all of their measurable tumors disappeared. Then he stopped treatment and followed the mice. Within months, about half of the mice developed recurrences and died. The remainder were cured.

So he had a 100 percent complete remission rate and a 50 percent cure rate. Then he began to reduce the doses of the drugs. He found that if he reduced the doses of the drugs by 20 percent, he still got a 100 percent complete remission rate. But he got only a 25 percent cure rate.

This was a very important experiment. He could see the folly of reducing doses of effective drugs in mice in a matter of weeks or months. In humans, it might take years to recognize that a lower dose produced poorer long-term results, even though the complete remission rate remained high. In most doctors' offices, it would never be noticed. If these mice were humans with metastatic cancer, reducing the dose would appear harmless as long as all the patients went into remission.

But just because you can't see tumor anymore doesn't mean it's all gone.

The holy grail of cancer treatment is to be able to find one cancer cell in a million normal cells—or a tumor marker that is present only when cancer cells are present. If you can't find any cells or the tumor marker, it most likely means the cancer is gone. Being able to accurately determine if there are any tumor cells present would revolutionize cancer treatment overnight. And if the cancer is gone, what do you do? Stop treatment, of course. If you could do this in the postoperative period, right after someone has had a tumor removed, you could select for adjuvant chemotherapy only those patients who needed it—and save the rest from unnecessary treatment. If you could do this after a patient had a complete remission, you could stop therapy at that point or know how long to keep going if the marker was still present.

But for most solid tumors, we don't have good tests for minimal residual disease. The only recourse is to stop treatment after a complete remission and wait to see how many people relapse before they reach the critical period for their tumor. But you have to get a complete remission first.

In fact, there is really only one cancer with a marker precise enough to guide treatment, and that is the rare tumor of the placenta, choriocarcinoma, which produces the gonadotropin hormone. Studies have shown the hormone is measurable when as few as a thousand cells are present. So when the hormone's level falls to zero, treatment can be stopped with confidence the patient is cured of cancer. While there has been considerable research in this area, finding similar markers in other, common tumors remains the holy grail.

The bone marrow cancer multiple myeloma is the most recent cancer to follow the pathway to complete remission, chronicity, and perhaps cure. Myeloma is a malignancy of plasma cells, the cells in the immune system that make our antibodies. Antibodies are our primary line of defense against bacterial infections. Plasma cells live in the bone marrow, so in a sense this is a cancer of the bone; malignant plasma cells generally don't circulate in the bloodstream in any quantity.

One of my notable experiences with this cancer came in the treatment of a patient named Mel Goldstein. I was director of Yale Cancer

Center at the time. He was the local weatherman on Channel 8 in New Haven. I used to watch his weather forecast at 6:00 in the morning while pumping away on my exercise bike. I have never seen Mel without a big toothy smile that went from ear to ear. He enjoyed weather—even bad weather—and the viewing public could sense this, and they felt good watching him.

I met Mel in 1996. He had developed acute back pain that was thought to be due to a slipped disk. It turned out there was a more sinister reason for his pain. Malignant plasma cells had accumulated in his vertebrae, making the bones so soft one had collapsed—a disturbing and extremely painful consequence of multiple myeloma.

At the time, myeloma was uniformly fatal, with a median survival of about forty-two months. Mel was about fifty when he was diagnosed. A median survival of less than four years didn't look good to him.

Although he was devastated by the diagnosis, he wanted to keep working. He went public on the air with his diagnosis early on and presented to the public a cheery view of a cancer patient few people had ever seen.

When he was diagnosed, the standard treatment was the use of two drugs, melphalan, a cousin of nitrogen mustard, the old war-gas derivative, and prednisone, a steroid. And that's what Mel got at first. There was nothing else approved for use. But while we were treating Mel, I got wind of two new classes of drugs that looked particularly promising in myeloma in early testing.

One was thalidomide, the infamous drug that inspired the FDA to tighten regulations in the 1960s. It had been resurrected as a potential anticancer drug, and there were hints it might work in myeloma. Mel wanted to try it. He became one of the earliest patients treated with it—and it worked.

The best myeloma program in the country is the one developed and run by my friend Ken Anderson, a professor at Harvard's Dana-Farber Cancer Institute. I told him what was going on with Mel. Ken was also developing more potent derivatives of thalidomide and had a few under test. He also had access to another new drug, bortezomib, that was in early testing by the Millennium pharmaceutical company. We had no access to these new drugs before FDA approval, but Ken did. I knew Yale couldn't catch up with what Ken was doing, and I told him so. "Can we piggyback on your program?" I said. He told me he would be happy to work with us.

You might hope that oncologists were concerned with the welfare of their patients most of all, but that's unfortunately not always the case. I had always made it a practice to refer patients to wherever the best work was going on for their disease. I found that most patients would move heaven and earth to take advantage of something that might save their lives. To meet requirements set by the drug's maker and the FDA, Ken would have to see Mel at Harvard. Everyone at Yale was against it. "It is too new to know if these drugs will work," they said. But most of all, they feared the negative publicity that might accompany sending such a well-known local figure as Mel Goldstein— one who talked openly about his treatment and where he got it—to another center. Especially Harvard. I made the arrangements anyhow, and Mel agreed not to publicize where he was getting treatment.

Mel Goldstein's case was another example of the importance of being around the action if you have a life-threatening disease. For this disease, the action was at Harvard, not Yale. He couldn't have known that, but he had me to serve as his advocate. If you can't be around the action, you need a good advocate to keep an eye out for where the action is, one willing to ignore traditional boundaries in medicine.

Mel kept a furtive eye on the pharmaceutical industry, hoping against hope that it would keep new drugs coming. He hoped that the FDA would permit him access to new drugs when he needed them, not when it deemed them ready. And he hoped the changes in the health-care system wouldn't lead to panels deciding that a new treatment, although it may extend a life, was not cost-effective.

Mel lived for sixteen years, cheerily chairing an annual survivors' luncheon, reminding everyone his tenure was supposed to have ended at forty-two months. "Help is on the way," he was fond of saying.

For a long time, the new drugs, one after another, controlled his disease. He lost a few inches in height as a result of his bone disease, and he walked with a cane. But he was spry on TV, and happy.

Today, we really don't know the median survival for myeloma patients. These developments are too new to have registered in the long-term survival data. But what happened with Mel is no longer unusual. Myeloma patients survive many years longer than the original forty-two-month median and survive in good shape, with a decent quality of life. Mel is unusual only in the sense that he got early access to treatments that now everyone can get.

Using these new drugs, combined with newly refined techniques of bone marrow transplantation, Ken Anderson and his group reported in 2010 that a large fraction of their patients with myeloma went into complete remission and appeared to stay there.[8] They might be cured. Time will tell. If so, they won't have a chronic disease anymore. I think of Mel when I read about these developments. We gave him extra years, and we came so close to giving him even more.

Early in the morning of August 10, 1813, British barges sailed up the Miles River off the Chesapeake Bay, intending to shell the town of St. Michaels and its harbor fort. The good people of St. Michaels, having been warned of the attack, ordered the populace to hang lanterns in the woods adjacent to the town and extinguish all the lights in the town itself, creating the first-ever wartime blackout.

The British spent the night shelling the woods. Only one stray cannonball hit a house near the fort in St. Michaels, known since then as Cannonball House. The motto of this story could be "Beware of shooting in the dark—you may not hit what you're aiming at."

For much of the twentieth century, chemotherapy was shooting in the dark. We knew where the town was—the DNA of the cancer cell—but we couldn't see well enough through the murk surrounding the DNA to target the cancer genes. So we fired in the general vicinity of the DNA, and occasionally, as in the case of Hodgkin's disease and acute lymphocytic leukemia, we got lucky. The cancers we cured with conventional combination chemotherapy were our cannonball houses—our somewhat improbable hits.

We are now in the age of what's called targeted chemotherapy. It's yet another paradigm shift. Unlike the older drugs that damaged DNA in nonspecific ways, targeted chemotherapy is aimed at specific molecular abnormalities that are, in many cases, unique to each cancer and uniquely involved in the cancer's growth. These targets are usually stations along the way in signaling pathways that involve cell growth or cell death. More often than not, the targets are genes that involve the hallmark of sustained proliferation signaling. So when you attack them, you can shut growth off, like switching off a lightbulb.

Or you can switch cell death on, which amounts to handing the cancer cell a sword and telling it to commit hara-kiri, thereby attacking another hallmark.

An important part of managing patients now is to do a genetic analysis of their tumor tissue to determine its molecular structure and find treatable mutations and then to select a treatment based on the mutations. This is the essence of personalized medicine. We are no longer shooting in the dark.

The best example is the treatment for chronic myeloid leukemia (CML), developed by my friend Brian Druker, the director of the Knight Cancer Institute at the Oregon Health and Science University. In the early 1970s, CML was incurable, and the average survival for CML was thirty-two months. The cancer went through a chronic phase and a phase of accelerated growth and finally ended in "blastic crisis," a phase indistinguishable from acute leukemia. The average age of onset was fifty-five, and with only a thirty-two-month median survival, patients did not live out their normal life spans.

My involvement with CML began in 1970 when George Canellos and I developed an improved treatment, using conventional combination chemotherapy, for blastic crisis. That extended survival to forty-eight months. Then we learned to use allogeneic bone marrow transplants (marrow from a matched, related donor) to replace the diseased marrow, which we could destroy with high doses of chemotherapy. Using this method, we could actually cure 25 percent of adults who had a related donor with a bone marrow match—usually from a matched sibling. There is only one chance in four that a sibling will be a match, and patients had to be under fifty and able to tolerate ablative marrow treatment, i.e., to destroy cancer in their own marrow. Most CML patients are over fifty, so the cure rate overall was very low. Then, in 2001, a new drug, Gleevec, arrived—a targeted chemotherapy agent. Researchers had discovered in the 1960s that CML arose from a particular genetic defect—the creation of a fusion gene called BCR-ABL that keeps the motor of CML cells running all the time. Gleevec shut that motor down.

Now we don't even know what the average life span is for this disease, because most people are living out a normal life span, in good health—as long as they take a pill every day. In most cases, they still have the molecular abnormality if you look hard enough for it. And in most cases, if you stop treatment, the cancer recurs. So it meets our definition of a chronic disease. However, unlike other metastatic cancers, the cancerous white blood cells in CML can perform the normal functions of white cells, so being defective doesn't matter. But after Gleevec, for all intents and purposes, the cancer is not visible anymore—to us and, more important, to the patients. The CML example proves that cancer can be converted to a chronic disease if you can find the right switch or switches to shut off.

But as you might suspect by now, that's not the end of the story. Cancer is too clever for that. After a while, CML cells in some patients learn how to get around Gleevec. They develop a mutation at the target site that Gleevec attacks, and that prevents the drug from binding and blocking that critical site. And the tumor no longer responds to Gleevec. But in a stroke of good luck for CML patients, the pharmaceutical industry has developed several new drugs to attack these new mutations at the target site. So with a switch to a new drug, these patients go on living a normal life. Most patients with CML keep an eye on the drug industry, hoping it will keep up with all the new mutations that can occur in CML cells. So far, it has.

There are also hints that these drugs can do more. If they are used in novel ways, they can destroy the entire diseased leukemic cell population. In some cases, after a complete remission with Gleevec, the molecular abnormality disappears, and the disease does not recur if the drug is stopped. We say these patients are cured "in all likelihood." In the near future, we may be able to cure CML entirely, but those we can't cure will have a near-normal life span, too. They will just need to continue taking medications. This is a kind of oncologist's nirvana.

As a test of targeted therapies, CML was easier to attack than other cancers. It is unique in having one dominant molecular abnormality. Most cancers have several. Cancer of the pancreas has twelve. In cancers with more than one abnormality, we will surely require combinations of targeted treatments and combination anti-hallmark therapy; that will be difficult to develop. But we have proof of principle that targeted chemotherapy works.

Another viable approach to attacking cancer cells is to induce senescence—make a cancer cell age, wear out, and die. There is a rare inherited disorder called Werner's syndrome in which affected patients are normal until puberty, when they start to age rapidly. It's the cellular equivalent of the picture of Dorian Gray—fast-track aging. People who have Werner's syndrome look seventy when they're forty.

We've actually identified some of the genes responsible for that extreme aging through studying cancer viruses, which need young cells to grow. These viruses have learned to block the proteins produced by senescence genes and to immortalize cells—to keep them young—so the cancer viruses and infected cells can keep growing. This happens when the papilloma virus infection of the cervix causes cervical cancer.

In patients with acute promyelocytic leukemia, which affects certain white blood cells, senescence is already the primary path to cure. An abnormal gene called RARA drives the growth of promyelocytic leukemia cells. RARA results from the fusion of two normal genes, one of which is the receptor for vitamin A (retinoic acid), a vitamin involved in cell maturation. Not only does RARA block the cells from aging, but it keeps the throttle down on growth, revving the cells up so that they'll divide frequently. That means lots of immortal cancerous cells. Not good. But we've discovered that by using vitamin A derivatives, we can target and confuse the errant genes. With one of these drugs, the white blood cells of patients with acute promyelocytic leukemia can mature again. Normal white cells live only about six days in circulation, so maturing them is very near killing them. In fact, one of the side effects of treatment with ATRA (all-trans retinoic acid, the first vitamin A derivative we used) is that the sudden load of mature white cells can clog up small blood vessels and cause difficulty breathing, fluid retention, and a host of other things.

We now have several of these vitamin A derivatives. By combining them and standard drugs for acute leukemia, we can drive most cells into very old age and kill those that don't mature. This once rapidly fatal disease is now curable about 70 percent of the time.

Dr. Stanley Cohen at Vanderbilt University was a basic scientist interested in cell growth. In the course of his experiments, he had injected newborn mice with extracts from salivary glands. He was surprised when the newborn mice prematurely opened their eyes and erupted teeth. Something in the salivary extracts was speeding cell growth.

He needed an assay system—a method of analysis—to be able to monitor the purification of a factor he had isolated from the salivary glands, which he called "tooth-lid factor." He was no stranger to these kinds of biologic assays. He had spent some time in 1953 at Washington University in St. Louis with another scientist, Rita Levi-Montalcini, isolating nerve growth factor, another material from salivary glands that stimulated nerve growth.

Ultimately, Cohen figured out that the material he was purifying was accelerating the growth and separation of epithelial cells that sealed the mouse eyelids and caused teeth to sprout. He discovered, isolated, purified, and sequenced a material he called epidermal growth factor (EGF), a protein that stimulates the growth of epithelial and other cells and enhances certain developmental growth.

He was also able to identify the target receptor for EGF and the mechanism of its action, providing a breakthrough in understanding how signals from outside a cell reach the inside of a cell, how cells talk to one another.

This turned out to be one of the most important discoveries of the twentieth century. It has had an important impact not only on the understanding of how cancers grow but also on cancer treatment. The discovery enabled scientists to further explore the cell growth process set in motion by EGF stimulation and to develop drugs to block the individual steps. The EGF receptor is expressed in virtually every cell in the body, and it is often over-expressed in cancer cells. This realization led to a huge increase in research on targeted therapies. In 1986, Cohen and Levi-Montalcini shared the Nobel Prize for identifying the first growth factors.

The biotech firm ImClone was one of the companies to take up the challenge of finding drugs to block EGF. I'm quite familiar with this work, because I was on the company's board when this research was being done. Researchers identified four EGF receptors—labeled EGF-1 through EGF-4. ImClone developed an antibody, called Erbitux, to block the EGF-1 receptor, the most common variety. The drug proved to be useful in prolonging survival in both colon and lung cancer patients. And its side effects on normal cells were trivial: a rash around hair follicles. (Oddly enough, people who got a rash responded to the drug more often than those who didn't.) Others discovered that EGF-2, also known as HER2, is over-expressed in about a third of patients with breast cancer. And it is not commonly expressed in normal cells. Another drug, Herceptin, which blocks the HER2 receptor, is a mainstay of the treatment of breast cancer.

In 2008, Tom Lynch, now the cancer center director at Yale, published a paper in *The New England Journal of Medicine* that identified a subset of lung cancer patients who had a mutation in the EGF receptor that made them sensitive to a new class of drugs that can inhibit a group of key enzymes involved in cell growth known as tyrosine kinases.[9] These kinases add phosphate groups to tyrosine residues in proteins, making the proteins a source of energy generation. They act primarily on the hallmark of sustained proliferation. Gleevec is also a kinase inhibitor. These new drugs can be given by mouth, like Gleevec. And several have also been approved for use in kidney cancer and primary cancer of the liver.

When the drugs were first studied in metastatic lung cancer, the results were negative. But a careful analysis of the data by Lynch and others showed that some studies, a small subset, were actually getting very good responses, far better than seen with older available drugs. And now several mutations have been discovered in patients with lung cancer—EGFR, discovered by Lynch himself, and two fusion genes known as EML4-ALK (ALK for short) and ROS1. All of them act to switch on growth when the signal should be the reverse. And for each mutation, we have a drug that works. For EGFR, we have two drugs, erlotinib and afatinib, that block these signals and produce good and sometimes long remissions, and for ALK and ROS1 we have two other drugs, crizotinib and ceritinib, that block the action of these fusion genes and produce good responses. Some of the drugs, in some patients, can even produce complete remissions.

The frequency of these mutations varies, depending on the makeup of the population, but in total rarely exceeds 20 percent of the lung cancer population. For example, they are more common in women, Asians, and nonsmokers. But identifying these mutations constitutes are the first major advance in lung cancer therapy in years.

Two things are certain. We will find more, and we know how to synthesize drugs to block not only the primary mutation but the mutations that lead lung cancer cells to become resistant to these drugs. There is a bright future here. All lung cancer patients should be screened for these mutations before treatment is started. If they have one, the treatment is effective and easier than standard chemotherapy, and they can be spared the toxicity of standard drugs.

The same thing has happened in metastatic melanoma, as I have noted in a previous chapter. Treatment with drugs that target a mutated gene, BRAF, found in about 60 percent of cases of melanoma, is producing quality remissions and prolonging life. Every success, such as this, has spurred further research. There are an increasing number of molecular targets being identified in cancer patients. So while current targeted therapy in tumors that occur in the lung and breast and colon is not yet as successful as Gleevec in CML, the future is bright for the use of combined targeted chemotherapy.

We can now cure more than 68 percent of all cancers—more if you count the easily curable skin cancers, which are very common. Frankly, in the long run, curing cancers may be easier than converting them into chronic diseases because the cancer cell is unique. Remember, cancer cells resemble cells in the early embryo, whose natural tendency is to divide like mad and make more cells—lots more cells. Embryonic cells have only nine months to make a baby; they must work very fast.

Generally, physicians are faced with an either-or situation when treating cancer. Either you remove the cancer with surgery; or you kill the cells with radiotherapy; or you use some form of systemic treatment in the bloodstream, like chemotherapy or immunotherapy, that gets everywhere. Otherwise, cancer cells will continue to divide. Whatever you do, if even a few cancer cells are left behind, you have to stop those cells from growing. For patients in whom we can't manage to remove all the cancer cells so they can live *with* their cancer, we will need to make cancer cells dormant—do something to them that just lets them sit there, not growing and not causing any problems. Or if they grow, we need to make them grow slowly—very slowly.

Is this doable? Has it ever happened? Yes, actually. There are circumstances in which cancers appear to stay dormant for long periods of time. These cases are intriguing, even though we have not been able to consistently reproduce them in other patients. Kidney cancer is one tumor that can do this, and because of this possibility, it sometimes warrants a different approach to the treatment of metastatic cancer.

Here's an example. Steve Rosenberg and I (we often work together managing patients' cases) took care of a colleague at the NIH. He had a kidney cancer removed and then developed pulmonary metastases, secondary deposits in his lungs, which are very common in kidney cancer. If there aren't too many, and if follow-up visits show that the growth rate is slow, they can be removed surgically.

At the time, Steve was working on what turned out to be a groundbreaking study treating kidney cancer using interleukin-2 (which spurs the growth of T lymphocytes) together with the patients' primed lymphocytes. But this was a new and highly experimental treatment. SW worried that it would be too much for him. Plus, his tumors met the criteria for surgical removal. Steve's group removed his metastases, and he stayed free of disease for several years. When his tumors recurred, again in the lungs, his doctors removed them again. With this approach, our colleague lived a pretty normal life for more than ten years. In as many as a quarter of the cases like this that are treated surgically, the tumor never recurs. The same approach can be taken in many sarcomas that metastasize to the lungs. Doctors sometimes forget about this in the rush to test new drugs. As a consultant, I often find myself reminding doctors of this too often overlooked way to convert some metastatic cancers into chronic diseases.

What can kidney cancer teach us that might prove useful to treating patients with other types of cancers? It had been noted, anecdotally, that some patients who present with kidney cancer that has already spread to their lungs go into a remission when you remove the primary tumor—the involved kidney.

This was once considered a rash thing to do. Why subject patients to expensive major surgery when they already had widespread cancer? There was no proof it worked, just the observation of a few overzealous (or very astute) doctors. In 2001, we did get some evidence in the form of two randomized controlled trials.[10] Half of patients who had a new diagnosis of metastatic kidney cancer were treated with interferon, a mediocre treatment for kidney cancer, while the other half were treated with removal of the diseased kidney plus interferon. In both studies, the survival of patients who had a kidney removed was significantly longer.[11]

What was the primary tumor doing to influence the growth of metastases? Can tumor cells talk to each other over great distances?

In 1889, the British surgeon Stephen Paget published a paper in *The Lancet* proposing what is referred to as the "seed and soil" hypothesis. He had noted a curious thing in patients who had died of breast cancer. There was a propensity for metastases to develop in the liver and bones over other sites. He said in that landmark paper, "The remote organs cannot be altogether passive or indifferent as regards metastases." In other words, the invaded organs are aware—or participate somehow—in the metastatic process.

He was right. We have long since figured out that specific tumors have preferred patterns of metastasis. But in 2005, 116 years after Paget's astute observation, experimental data by a group of researchers from Weill Cornell Medical Center provided an explanation to confirm that an organ next on the list for invasion is, in fact, a participant in the metastasis.[12] The study showed that there was communication between the primary tumor and preferred sites of metastases. It demonstrated that the primary cancer summons cells from the bone marrow to the tumor's preferential sites of metastases to prepare a "pre-metastatic niche"—a nest, if you will, that makes the sites hospitable for invasion by the errant cancer cells. Without that preparation, metastases cannot acquire the hallmarks they need to survive and grow.

My colleague Larry Norton has also done some fine work that shows prostate cancer cells will migrate back to the prostatic bed after a primary tumor has been removed. Why? Probably they like the environment and find it favorable for acquiring all the hallmarks of cancer. This has led to the use of postoperative radiation of the surgical site to control prostate cancer.

Since this work, other researchers have identified specific chemicals that primary tumors secrete to set up these niches. Their interest piqued, other scientists have begun to look at the influence of removal of the primary tumor—the instigator, it seems—in other types of metastatic cancers. So far, it seems that in breast cancer, and probably prostate cancer, this remote signaling is an active phenomenon.

In the early 1970s, when I was chief of medicine at the NCI, I saw a forty-nine-year-old perimenopausal patient with breast cancer. She was the wife of a prominent science administrator at the NIH, so I was asked to take care of her personally. She had already had a radical mastectomy elsewhere a few years earlier, and because the lymph glands under her arm had been found to have cancer cells in them, she had been put on adjuvant chemotherapy. But that hadn't worked, and now the cancer had appeared in her lungs and abdomen. She had exhausted all the available drugs and was in bad shape.

Further, I'd met her socially when she was with her husband, a gruff, in-your-face kind of guy with a deep bass voice and big shocks of unruly, curly white hair. He didn't like what we were doing at the NCI, and he tried to get her away from us, as sick as she was. He was a typical data-driven, skeptical scientist, and he gave me heat about doing anything further without "evidence" that it might help her. I really felt like asking him why he hadn't brought her in sooner, because we did have data on how to treat such patients if we saw them earlier.

She had been admitted to a private room in the NIH Clinical Center on another service that didn't ordinarily admit cancer patients. When I first walked into her room, I saw a woman who hardly resembled the one I had met at social events. She was emaciated, pale, and deeply distressed. It was a depressing sight, exacerbated by the colorless, depressing room with government-green metal walls and green-and-black floor tiles. Her abdomen had been drained of fluid several times, and the repeated punctures had caused an infection, so she was on multiple antibiotics.

She had what we called the six-tube sign—six different bottles were hanging over her, with lines running into veins in her arms and legs. She also had a tube in her nose to decompress her stomach. As residents, we used to say if a patient had the six-tube sign, death was not too far behind. She was having trouble breathing, and her abdomen was swollen. Her blood pressure was unstable, and there was a question of whether or not we should just let her go. But she wasn't ready to give up. "Dr. DeVita, am I going to die?" she said. I told her what she already knew. "You're not in good shape, but we'll do everything we can to prevent you from dying."

At her stage of illness, there was little in the way of treatments that had been tested and found to be effective. I was operating in the never-never land of no data. But if there is any chance of a good outcome, I like to give the patient the benefit of the doubt. The fact that she was perimenopausal complicated things. Hormones can sometimes be a useful treatment, but we don't know whether they are effective in women her age. She had never been treated with hormones, and it was difficult to know whether we should add hormones or try to take them away.

So I suggested we irradiate her belly, because we might accomplish two things at the same time: slowing down the fluid formation from her tumor, and wiping out her ovaries. If her ovaries were still producing enough estrogen to drive her tumor growth, knocking them out with radiation might result in an antitumor effect by depriving the tumor of estrogen, which was driving the hallmark proliferation. At the least, I didn't think it would make her situation worse.

Her husband didn't like the idea. "It sounds like you're grasping at straws," he protested. "I am," I said. The radiotherapist didn't like the idea, either. It was very difficult to get her to the radiation therapy facility and treat her with all the tubes coming out of her body, and both the radiotherapist and her husband thought it futile anyhow. But she wanted it done, and her husband grudgingly agreed.

The radiation slowed the fluid formation pretty quickly, and over a period of several weeks her infection went away. In a month, the tumors in her lungs disappeared. We looked very hard to find the tumor in her abdomen, but that was gone, too.

Six weeks after being near death's door, she went home, with no more treatment required. I saw her regularly in the clinic as the years went by, but we never treated her with anything again. I was afraid to. I didn't know quite why she had responded so brilliantly and I didn't want to rock the boat. She led a normal life. We weren't sure what had happened or why the radiation made such a dramatic difference. But each of these cases is something we can learn from. The doubting oncologists would never have treated this woman. But to me, people are not cases. Each person has a life, a family, a future—and the right to whatever we can do.

Ten years later, her tumor came roaring back in the same places it had been before. This time, however, it was totally unresponsive to any chemotherapy or further hormone management, and she died in a very short period of time. It was an aggressive tumor before I saw her and just as aggressive, if not more so, when it grew back. In between, it was dormant for ten untroubled years.

Some years later, I was called by a former trainee of mine, Charles "Mick" Haskell, out in Los Angeles, about another patient with metastatic breast cancer. Mrs. W. was in her late sixties. She'd had a mastectomy, but the cancer had recurred and metastasized to her bones and lungs. She was postmenopausal, the right age to try hormone treatment, and bone involvement often responds to it. But over the phone, he told me he'd already tried it, and she hadn't responded. He now wanted to put her on the chemotherapy drug Adriamycin, which was a standard of care at the time. But there was a hitch. Adriamycin causes hair loss. Mrs. W. was a prominent, wealthy Beverly Hills socialite. She didn't like the idea of losing her hair, so she refused to take the drug.

Haskell pleaded for a special favor. "Vince," he said, "all I want you to do is come see her and reaffirm that she should go on Adriamycin. She needs an authority figure to reinforce my recommendation." She was an important patient to him, so I agreed to fly out and serve as a consultant.

When I arrived at the Los Angeles airport, I got a hint as to why Mrs. W. was so important to Mick Haskell. Out front, a chauffeur stood next to a cream-colored 1932 Rolls-Royce Silver Cloud classic.

He was holding a card with my name on it, and he was waiting to take me to the Beverly Wilshire hotel, where Mrs. W. and her daughter each owned a luxurious apartment. Then, he informed me, he was to take me to see Mrs. W. at the clinic and squire me around Beverly Hills. I should have been pleased, I suppose. But the lavish handling was merely making me feel guilty about coming to L.A. with nothing more to offer Mrs. W. than *Yes, I agree, you should go on Adriamycin.*

Later that afternoon, at the hospital, I asked to review Mrs. W.'s chart and her X-rays before I went into the clinic room to examine her. Within five minutes, I saw something that Haskell had missed. Mrs. W. was not hormone unresponsive. The hormone treatment had produced a flare-up of her disease, and new bone lesions had appeared on her X-ray exams, leading them to think she was getting worse. So they'd stopped treatment. But it's not unusual for invisible bone metastases to become visible when tumor in bone begins to respond to treatment. The involved bone around the tumor begins to remodel itself, and thinned-out areas affected by tumor infiltration, which had been too small for detection, then light up even on plain X-rays. Mrs. W.'s X-rays showed that she was, in fact, very sensitive to hormones.

I called Mick over. "Putting her on Adriamycin is the wrong thing to do," I told him, and I explained what I thought was going on. "I think she should go back on hormone therapy." We could easily manage any flare-ups with other drugs. Best of all, she would have few side effects, and she would not lose her hair. Haskell, who is a superb physician, was mortified at having missed a basic diagnosis. I reminded him that it happens to the best of us, and it had happened to me.

When I introduced myself to Mrs. W. and examined her, I could see why she had bucked at the idea of losing her hair due to a treatment that might only extend her life for a few more months at most. She looked quite elegant, even in a hospital gown, with carefully coiffed hair. She was delighted with my recommendation. And she was happy with Mick, too, for suggesting I come and see her. We treated her, and she went into a complete remission. All of her bone lesions healed, and her lung metastases cleared. And she stayed in remission.

Every time I went to Los Angeles to see her, she put the Rolls at my disposal. "Drive it yourself," she said. "Not on your life," I replied. I did, however, accept her offer to stay at the Beverly Wilshire hotel, a wing and a few floors away from her apartments. Mrs. W. lived to see her daughter marry, and she saw two grandchildren born and raised before her tumor recurred ten years later, at the age of seventy-eight. When it came back, it was aggressive, and it killed her in a matter of months.

Both my colleague's wife and Mrs. W. had aggressive cancers that had been growing rapidly. And in both cases, we'd been able to put them in a state of dormancy for at least a decade. By tinkering with their hormone pathways, we had reset the growth mechanisms of these remaining cancer cells—shut them off, so to speak. I suspect we in-activated a driver hallmark without which the cells couldn't grow. Or inactivated some aspect of the microenvironment that was vital to tumor growth.

Another hallmark of cancer, you might recall, is the ability to induce angiogenesis—that is, the ability to trigger the formation of new blood vessels to bring nutrients to a tumor. This, too, offers us an opportunity to stop cancer's growth. Deny it nutrients, and a tumor will shrink and either die or remain dormant. The researcher who did some of the landmark work in this area was Judah Folkman, a professor, a pediatric surgeon, and an outstanding laboratory investigator at Harvard.

Folkman, who died in 2008, was a delightful person. Everyone liked Judah. Of modest height and a soft build, he had the air of a schmoozer. He was the kind of guy you wanted to go out and have a beer with. In the 1960s, well before we knew about the hallmarks of cancer, he got the idea that tumors must help themselves grow by making their own blood vessels—to be sure they got the nourishment they needed. If this was true, then they had to make factors that stimulated blood vessels to grow to the tumor. "Angiogenic factors," he called them. If he could stop the angiogenesis, maybe he could starve the tumor to death. So he began what became a four-decade-long search for angiogenic factors.

His animal model was blood vessel growth in the eye of a rabbit, because it was easy to visualize. He would add extracts from tumors to rabbits' eyes to see whether the extracts caused blood vessels to grow.

While everyone liked and trusted Judah, no one believed the work was important in the beginning. When I was a clinical associate at the NCI, we used to go to the big clinical meetings, then held in Atlantic City, New Jersey, where Judah made presentations almost every year. It was kind of a joke. Doctors in the audience actually made fun of him. He could isolate something he called the angiogenic factor, but he couldn't purify it. Each year he showed us a dark blur on a chromatographic plate. Over time, the blur kept getting sharper and sharper. He was getting closer and closer to isolating the growth factor. While others joked, Judah persevered, and his persistence paid off.

When he finally isolated and described angiogenic factors, he was venerated for having opened an entirely new field of cancer treatment. He then identified agents that blocked the angiogenic factors. These angiogenesis blockers were called angiostatin and endostatin. And he suggested that the dormancy in the patient cases I've just described was possibly due to surviving tumor cells that were too far from blood vessels to get the needed nourishment to divide.

To test his factors against actual cancers, he needed another animal model. He chose the mouse. He injected human tumor cells into the skin of mice and then he injected the mice with his anti-angiogenic factors.

The tumors invariably shrank to nothing. He also showed that if you biopsied the mouse skin, there were a few surviving tumor cells trying their best to get as close to blood vessels as they could to get nourishment. They were alive but not growing.

And here is the startling thing about Judah's experiments: The mice lived normally as long as you continued treatment. They never developed resistance to anti-angiogenic factors, something that regularly defeats ordinary anticancer drugs. Here was the dormancy factor we had been looking for.

Judah was so sure he had found a new way to cure cancer that he told his graduate students and his assistants that he would double the salary of anyone who could find a tumor type that did not respond in his model. None did.

Judah won many prizes, including the Lasker prize, for his work. Many thought the Nobel Prize was sure to follow. Bristol-Myers Squibb was so excited about the results that it invested $40 million for the rights to develop angiostatin.

On Sunday, May 3, 1998, a front-page story by Gina Kolata of *The New York Times* extolled these compounds in such exuberant language that the stock in EntreMed—the company Judah formed to develop these compounds for clinical use—rose from $12 a share to $85 a share the next day. It helped that the Nobel laureate Jim Watson, one of the discoverers of the structure of DNA, told the *Times* that "Judah will cure cancer within two years."

The exuberance and excitement didn't last. There soon were reports that others were not able to repeat the work in Judah's lab and that Bristol-Myers Squibb was having trouble reproducing the experiments with angiostatin as well. This was confirmed in February 1999, when the company announced it was discontinuing its angiostatin research program. Goodbye to that $40 million.

I attended a think-tank meeting in Aspen, Colorado, in September 1999 hosted by the billionaire investor and philanthropist Ted Forstmann. It was a wide-open debate, and it was fun. We discussed everything from banking to medicine. I was on a panel with Craig Venter, the scientist who was a pioneer in the sequencing of the human genome, and other prominent scientists. Looking at the audience was like looking at a who's who of celebrities. Oprah Winfrey, Colin Powell, Martha Stewart, Dick Cheney, and a whole host of other celebrities were sitting right in front of us. We were describing what was hot and what was not, and when anti-angiogenesis came up, I mentioned the difficulty researchers had had repeating Judah Folkman's work.

Jim Watson was in the audience and rose to his feet to speak. He said he wasn't worried about Judah's data; others would soon replicate them. And then he repeated his blockbuster prediction. "Two years ago, I said that Judah Folkman would cure cancer within two years," he told the attendees. "I was wrong. But he will do it in another two years."

The audience was stunned. So was I. The Nobel Prize gives you a lot of credibility, and I could see the look on people's faces as they digested Watson's comment. Judah presented his work at the meeting of the American Society of Clinical Oncology in a plenary session the following year. The place was mobbed. Judah stood far away, high up on a stage, while his giant image was projected on big screens everywhere to an audience that numbered more than ten thousand doctors. I tried to raise a question from a floor microphone to address some concerns I had, but in the pandemonium I couldn't even get heard.

That was fifteen years ago. While neither angiostatin nor endostatin ever panned out, other compounds that inhibit tumor blood vessel growth did make it to the market. The foremost was bevacizumab (Avastin). Some of these drugs are effective in prolonging the life of cancer patients—but only for a few months. Not years—certainly not for a normal life span. The drugs are nowhere near as effective in practice as they were in Folkman's mouse experiments. Not enough, for sure, to convert cancer into a chronic disease.

The excitement over anti-angiogenesis was a measure of oncologists' desire to take a new and different path. And the results did not support the enthusiasm. What went wrong? Was Judah being dishonest?

There were whispers to that effect, but I couldn't believe it. Judah Folkman was one of the most decent, honest scientists I had ever met, and I felt his integrity was beyond reproach.

As it turned out, he was blinded by the thought of seeing his work reach fruition. As a consequence, he didn't see the defect in his experiments. He tested his chemicals against a whole variety of human tumors—breast cancers, colon cancers, sarcomas, and more. They all shrank to nothing. And they all had been implanted in the skin of a mouse.

Ultimately, the research showed that the target of angiostatin was the normal blood vessel in the mouse skin—not the tumor. Judah had proved that angiostatin worked very effectively on the blood vessels of the mouse skin. And that's all. We don't have mouse skin. And the tumors that kill our patients are not in skin; they are in the lungs and liver and other organs nourished by their own human blood vessels. If I worked for Judah Folkman, I could have doubled my salary by changing the design of his experiment. I tried to tell him this, but he wouldn't listen. I mentioned it to some of his close friends, hoping he might listen to them. And I was scoffed at. The implication that somehow Judah was wrong was unacceptable.

Judah's work did provide proof of principle that you could starve tumors to death or put them in a dormant state if you shut down their blood supply. But mice are not people. Though mice can be useful proxies at times, everything that happens in them is not necessarily replicated in humans. You need to seriously evaluate what happens in a mouse before you conclude that it will be the same in humans.

Shutting down a tumor's blood supply remains a viable approach to cancer treatment. A deficient blood supply might explain why some tumors remain dormant for years, as in the cases I described. But used by themselves, anti-angiogenic compounds haven't yet been able to convert cancer into a chronic disease, as Judah hoped. As we all hoped. They might do that yet. We just haven't yet learned how best to exploit them. But there is good evidence that they will need to be used in combination with other anti-hallmark treatments to reach their potential.

What the field is now ablaze with are the exciting results manipulating another hallmark of cancer: normal immune surveillance. Steve Rosenberg was the first to actively research whether the immune system is capable of responding to cancer. Most had assumed no, because cancer seemed to run wild, untreated, unimpeded by the immune system's tools for attacking foreign invaders. The assumption was that because cancer cells arose from our own bodies, our immune systems failed to recognize them.

But in 1968, when Rosenberg was a young doctor at the West Roxbury VA hospital, he met a patient who, at least for him, challenged that assumption. The patient showed up with a gallbladder problem. When Rosenberg checked the man's medical records, he found that the man, whom he refers to as DeAngelo, had been sent home to die twelve years earlier. He had been, according to the records, riddled with cancer. Yet here he was, in for a routine gallbladder problem, having received no treatment for the cancer that everyone had assumed had long since killed him.

Rosenberg believed DeAngelo's immune system had done it. But how, and why in him and not others? This was the beginning of what turned out to be Rosenberg's lifelong quest to establish that the human immune system was capable of recognizing and responding to cancer, and to amp up its abilities to make the effect stronger. In 1985, Rosenberg published an article in *The New England Journal of Medicine* showing that a small fraction of patients with melanoma and kidney cancer responded to an infusion of their lymphocytes jazzed up by a growth factor that stimulated their growth. But while some of these responses were brilliant, most patients didn't respond, despite years of tinkering with the system.

For decades, attempts at immunotherapy fell short of what we expected. Some researchers went back to the earlier, pessimistic stance with regard to the immune system's capacity to respond to cancer. But this changed with Jim Allison's discovery, in 1996, of the importance of immune checkpoints, a mechanism within cells that acts as a barricade capable of shutting down the immune system and preventing it from reacting against our own bodies.[13]

Our lymphocytes are normally useful in fighting foreign invaders, but they would be harmful if they attacked normal cells. They don't do that, because Mother Nature put a system in place in normal cells to shut them down, to keep them from damaging normal tissue. Cancer cells also possess this ability and use it to shut the immune system out if it recognizes them as foreign.

Two of the checkpoints, known as CTLA4* and PD-1, have been identified, and we've learned to disable them with drugs, allowing killer lymphocytes to see cancer cells and recognize them as rogue cells that need to be annihilated. Two of these drugs have been approved somewhat tardily by the FDA, and approval of another should come soon. And there must be at least twenty checkpoint blockers in development. We are seeing astonishing responses with them, so far, in melanoma and non-small-cell lung cancer, a common killer. Patients with these cancers are now hovering between a chronic disease state and an outright cure. Here's an interesting point. Every lung cancer doctor I know now feels that the anti-PD-1 drugs are, hands down, the best available treatment for metastatic lung cancer—but only those on clinical trials are getting access to them. Two of these drugs have been approved by the FDA for melanoma, and though we know the safety profile for them because of the melanoma studies, they have not yet been approved for lung cancer. Thousands of patients with lung cancer are being deprived of years of good life, right now, for no earthly reason.

---

*My friend Lee got an early version of the anti-CTLA4 antibody at the NCI. He developed side effects, and the treatment was stopped. I have often thought about his unusually good response to chemotherapy after that and wondered if it was in part due to delayed effects of anti-CTLA4 therapy.

In addition to all this, Steve Rosenberg, who never gave up on the idea of boosting patients' own cells, has pioneered the genetic engineering of patients' own killer T lymphocytes.[14] Rosenberg's technique allows him to remove the cells from the patient and arm them, in the lab, to attack any marker or mutation on any cancer cell when reintroduced to the patient.[15] Again, the early results in patients who have exhausted all treatments and are near death have been astonishing. Those who have seen the responses believe we have finally arrived at the point where immunotherapy has reached its full potential.

An interesting phenomenon is associated with these agents. Some cancer patients are slow to respond to them, and their response can be stretched out over a long period of time. What's more, their tumors may never completely disappear. It appears as if the immune system is stopping the tumor's growth but not entirely destroying it. These patients can see significant prolongation of life without going into complete remission—until now the sine qua non of curing cancer.

We now have something beneficial to offer for virtually every patient with metastatic cancer. We can sometimes manage widespread cancers in such a way that they behave like chronic diseases, even if the cancer remains visible. Or we can put cancer cells into a dormant state. Or we can use targeted chemotherapy, if we have a target and a drug that blocks that target, to convert an increasing number of cancers into a chronic state.

But combination targeted chemotherapy or combination anti-hallmark therapy offers the most hope for the death of cancer if we can learn to harness it effectively and apply it to patients in a personalized way. Doing that requires more than science; it requires enough flexibility to outsmart the cancer cell.

Mary Lasker made two tactical errors when she launched the war on cancer. The first was that she misjudged the effect of promising a terrified public a cure in an impossible time frame.

The second was in thinking that being able to cure advanced cancer with drugs meant we had reached critical mass. We hadn't. Winston Churchill, in reference to a victory claimed by the Allies in North Africa, once said, "Now this is not the end. It is not even the beginning of the end. But it is, perhaps, the end of the beginning." In 1972, we were at the very most at the end of the beginning. Now I believe we are at true critical mass—the beginning of the end.

11

In 2009, I received another one of those calls that someone had cancer. This time, the patient was me.

I've been running a mile or two a day for decades without incident. Since we moved to Connecticut, when I went to Yale, my route has consisted of a two-mile loop to the end of our road and back. In the winter of 2006, while running this route, I slipped on a piece of black ice. It caused just enough of a jolt to tear a piece of cartilage in my right knee.

Doctors can be quirky when it comes to their own health. Some conscientiously get annual physicals, eat well, and exercise regularly. Others assiduously avoid doctor's appointments and completely ignore the advice they regularly hand out to patients.

I knew a surgeon with the ironic name Brian Blades. As a resident, he'd scrubbed in with Evarts Graham, who performed the first operation to remove a lung as treatment for lung cancer. Blades went on to become a well-known lung cancer surgeon himself, although he used to break scrub during operations to go have a smoke. This, even though he'd held lungs half decayed from cancer in his hands. He died of lung cancer.

I fall somewhere in the middle as far as inadvisable physician behavior. I've always eaten pretty well. When the research made it clear that fruit, vegetables, and fiber were helpful in preventing heart disease, and maybe cancer, I changed my diet. I smoked for a time, until the surgeon general's report on smoking and health provided evidence linking tobacco and cancer. I've always exercised regularly.

My physician's vice was that I had always avoided going to the doctor. For anything. I behaved this way for the same reason many people who avoid doctors do: I'm afraid of bad news. In my case, I can imagine a little too clearly the form that news might take.

Avoiding medical care, of course, takes a certain degree of forbearance. It means tolerating a certain degree of pain and discomfort. I'd learned that I could ignore and put up with a lot, over the years. But in 2006, the pain and swelling in my knee was too bad to ignore. I had no choice but to go to an orthopedist and have it looked at. And when a scan revealed a meniscal tear and medical therapy didn't work, I had no choice but to agree to surgery.

My recovery was complicated by urinary retention, which means the bladder does not want to empty. It's a common enough postsurgical complication. In me, it was worse, because I had an enlarged prostate gland that I had assiduously avoided any medical care for. Why? Because the symptoms and signs of an enlarged prostate gland and prostate cancer are similar. My deepest fear was that I had prostate cancer. In the wake of my surgery and its complications, however, there was no way to avoid the question. And now a new horror was before me. If my symptoms were due to cancer, I'd been ignoring them for a long time. It could be very advanced.

The doctor I saw to relieve the retention was no dummy. He looked at me, sitting in a flimsy blue gown on a hard metal examining table, obviously very anxious, and said, "You should have a PSA." "No," I replied. But I agreed to let him do a manual exam.

You can tell a lot by the feel of the prostate gland. A normal gland feels smooth and pliable. Lumps and hard edges are bad, a sign that something abnormal has transformed the tissue. As the doctor did my exam, I mentally ran through it with him, as if I were doing it myself, almost feeling the hard edge of the gland with my own fingertips. I braced myself for the bad news.

"It feels normal," he said.

I nearly cried with relief. "You really should have a TURP, though," he said.

TURP is short for "transurethral resection of the prostate," in which a portion of the enlarged prostate is removed in order to relieve pressure on the bladder. I should have had it years before. But I hadn't even considered it. To have a TURP, I'd have had to address the issue of whether cancer was involved. Now that my mind had been eased on that point, I felt I could go ahead with it.

I had the procedure and felt better than I had in years, especially with the nagging fear of cancer resolved. I took it as a cautionary tale. I resolved not to ignore health problems any longer. I not only found a primary care physician; I found one who wasn't intimidated by me. With his help, I began checking off a number of minor issues I'd failed to attend to over the years.

When I started having prostate symptoms again, two years later, I chalked them up to scar tissue from the original TURP. Not that unusual. At my annual visit with my urologist, he told me I'd need a mild procedure to trim it out. I went to my family doctor to have the blood work and checkup required before surgery. Unbeknownst to me, he ran a PSA, along with my other blood work. It came back at 10.8. High.

Needless to say, I was shocked. Now my surgeon would be on a dual mission—to remove scar tissue and to do a biopsy. Within a few days, I had the news—cancer. It only got worse from there. I got a call from my urologist. "Vince, the Gleason score is *neiynnee*," he said, garbling the number. He had a hard time getting the number out, because he knew what he was telling me. This was no slow-growing, something-else-will-kill-you-first prostate cancer. Just like Lee's, it appeared to be a bad actor.

You might assume that with my background, and at this point in my career, I would know exactly what to do and whom to go to. You might assume that I wouldn't be completely bowled over, to the point of numbness, by my diagnosis. But you would be wrong.

For close to a week, I lived in a daze. What ran repetitively through my head were the various scenarios that would take place leading to my death. I knew them all; I'd seen them happen. It had happened to Lee. This is the curse of being a doctor who gets ill, and the double curse of being a doctor who gets a disease from his own field.

I had always been a champion for my patients and never left a stone unturned looking for new approaches. But for me it was different. I didn't want to look at the literature, because I had a good idea of what I would see.

Meanwhile, I worried about the news getting out. I canceled several of my commitments at the annual meeting of the American Society of Clinical Oncology. I never miss ASCO meetings, so my absence would be notable. I fretted that rumors would start to fly. For years, I'd given the image of being indestructible. I didn't want to appear vulnerable. I knew, however, that the news would get out eventually, and I dreaded it.

After about a week of this, one thing did become clear to me. I was susceptible to all the same things Lee had been, including cookbook medicine and nonaggressive care. But while I had steered countless people through the potential obstacles over the course of my career, I didn't think I had the wherewithal to do it for myself. I couldn't be my own advocate, nor did I want to be. But who could? For my entire career as an oncologist, I'd worried about this. I always thought if I got cancer, I needed a Jay Freireich to take care of me. Someone who would go the extra mile. But Jay was not the answer. This was not his field, and he was no longer seeing patients anyhow.

And I had another complication. I am not a celebrity in the world at large, but in my own field, oncology, I'm well known. That was bad, not just because it made me feel exposed, but because celebrities, notoriously, get the worst medical care. People cut corners for a celebrity's convenience, and something bad often happens. Look what happened to Joan Rivers. Apparently, so that she could avoid the attention of being admitted to a hospital, the usual safeguards were ignored, and it cost her. I could probably talk a doctor into doing something foolish, too.

Finally, the answer became obvious to me. I needed Steve Rosenberg, chief of surgery at the NCI. Prostate cancer was not his field either, but Steve is an excellent clinician with a keen searching mind, and I knew how devoted he was to his patients. Steve and I had been friends since my early days at the NCI. His work consisted of not only performing fine surgery but painstakingly pioneering the new field of immunotherapy to treat cancer, a field that has now led to the cure of a significant fraction of patients with advanced melanoma and a new and exciting approach to advanced cancers using genetically engineered T cells.

Steve and I had been co-editors on a cancer textbook for years and had spent a lot of time together. He was the kind of doctor who would advocate for you, who would try everything. I'd seen him race into IRB meetings, white coat flying behind him, fire in his eyes, to ask for protocol amendments that IRBs are usually reluctant to grant. He usually got them. He was the kind of doctor you wanted. He was the kind of doctor, specifically, that I wanted to navigate for me.

I e-mailed him, and he answered immediately, asking for the details of my case. There was no doubt that it was a tricky one. My prostate gland was unusually large; the PSA and Gleason score were both high. Odds were that the cancer had metastasized. The standard of care in that scenario was radiation and hormone therapy. We both knew that in my case this wouldn't give me much of a shot. By now, I had had both a CT scan and an MRI. They both confirmed a very large prostate gland, but the good news was that there was no evidence the tumor had spread beyond the gland.

Steve got on the phone and started calling surgeons across the country. He shared my records but avoided using my name so people would not make a special exception for the former NCI director. The results were gloomy. One of the best-known and pioneering prostate surgeons in the country told Steve that if I were his case, he wouldn't operate on me even if I had no metastases. The prostate gland was too large, he said. He recommended radiotherapy.

My Yale surgeon, too, was reluctant to operate due to the size of the prostate gland. He recommended that I see a Yale radiotherapist who specialized in prostate cancer treatment. I did. It was one of the most discouraging hours I have ever spent. He was brutal. More so, I think, than he would have been for the average patient. He said he could irradiate me but, because of the gland size, the results would be horrendous. In addition to not controlling the tumor, the radiation would cause disabling side effects to my urinary tract. He went on to describe them, in minute detail, emphasizing over and over again the utter hopelessness of my case. Then he went to call in the house staff to examine me. But I just got up and walked out. Because the surgeons were not happy operating, and the radiotherapists were not inclined to irradiate the gland, that left hormone therapy. That was a straight line to death for a case like mine.

Steve's calls had led him to believe that my best option was to see Peter Scardino, a surgeon at MSKCC. Now I had two new problems. Though I'd gone through the early process of the diagnosis at Yale, I was pretty sure that I wanted to follow Steve's advice and have surgery at MSKCC rather than at my own institution. I had an excellent surgeon at Yale. I had helped recruit him ten years earlier, in fact, but he too was reluctant to operate, and Yale had no real urologic team to back him up. The management of major cancers is a team approach. All the specialties need to get involved at the outset to plan the entire course of treatment for the patient. My experience with our radiotherapist, with his blunt assessment of my chances (possibly affected by who I was), told me I didn't want him involved. And Yale had no medical oncologist at the time who specialized in prostate cancer. MSKCC was full of specialists in all these areas. It had my good

longtime friend Zvi Fuks as chief of radiotherapy as well as Howard
Scher, a medical oncologist and one of the leading prostate cancer
doctors in the country. And they had an excellent team behind them.

I had a frank talk with my Yale urologist. He was great about it,
admitting that he was a bit alone, and lamented the difficulty he was
having building a team. He also said I should explore MSKCC for
another reason—privacy. While he would do everything possible to
keep my case private, he said, we both knew that everything that
happened to me would be all over the hospital in minutes.

In the end, Steve and I agreed that the best place for me was
MSKCC. It had the top oncology team for prostate cancer in the country, he felt. Scardino was highly recommended by everyone Steve spoke
to as a technically excellent surgeon. He only did open procedures, no
laparoscopes, no robotics. Others in the department were using the
da Vinci robot. But because of the size of my prostate gland, I was not
a candidate for that.

Scardino agreed to see me. I called my friend Zvi Fuks, who would
squire me through the additional workup they would do. Sloan Kettering didn't accept test results from other institutions, especially
MRIs, an area in which machine quality was changing rapidly. I'd
have to have another round of scanning there. Sloan Kettering had
a more sophisticated MRI machine than Yale's, with a much more
powerful magnet, so they could see tissue in more detail. And it was
used with a special rectal coil to further increase the sensitivity. This
one showed a signal—a hot spot, if you will—in an area of some pelvic
lymph nodes and possibly nearby bone. It looked as if the cancer had
spread, after all. This, beyond terrifying me, was a potential wrench in
the plans. Most places wouldn't operate on someone in my position, in
which it appeared the cancer had spread not only to nodes but maybe
to pelvic bones. But that, we all knew, left me absolutely no chance.

Because the MRI I'd had at Sloan Kettering was done with an
experimental machine, it wasn't impossible that the results were a
false positive. I returned home and met once more with my Yale surgeon. His suggestion was that we attempt to do a needle biopsy of

the "hot" areas to determine if the lymph nodes were positive. If the biopsy was negative, we could go ahead and attempt the surgery. He said he wouldn't want to undertake such big surgery without the biopsies.

I didn't like the idea of someone fishing around my pelvis with a needle, and I was uncomfortable with his reluctance to operate. I called Steve again. "Vince, go to Peter Scardino," he said. "Your surgeon is going to have to be a warrior to do this operation, and you don't want a reluctant warrior." He was right.

Scardino was in a tough position. If the scan was right and he did the surgery, he could be criticized for being too aggressive, especially if something happened to me during the operation. If he didn't operate and the scan was wrong, I might have lost my best chance at survival.

Zvi agreed that radiotherapy just wasn't in the cards. In the end, Scardino decided to brave any potential negative blowback he would get from his own operative review board, ignore the results of the MRI, and go ahead with the surgery. In other words, he was going to go the extra mile for me. Doing the surgery would get me from a zero chance to be cured to 50 percent if it was successful. Not a small difference. It was my only chance.

On May 19, 2009, I walked into MSKCC, shed my watch and my ring, and donned the traditional surgical gown. As I drifted in and out of consciousness in the recovery room, Scardino's pathologist was busy looking at the frozen sections of the tissue to see if tumor was present.

At first pass, the lymph nodes looked clean. Now I would have to wait a week for the final review of the tissue.

I spent six days in the hospital. On May 26, I went home to recuperate and to await the final pathology results, which would tell me if the tumor had metastasized.

Paralyzed with anxiety, I ripped through an unseemly number of mystery novels—the most effective way I had of disengaging my mind from the worry. Every time the anxiety surfaced, every time I woke up in the middle of the night, I picked up a book in an attempt to stave off the indecision and uncertainty about the next step. One week from surgery, Peter called.

"Vince, I have very good news. All the lymph nodes are negative." The MRI was probably picking up a signal from a reactive lymph node there as a consequence of my prior surgery. Lymph nodes swell sometimes if there is inflammation around them. "And," he said, "in reviewing the MRI, they don't think there was a bone signal, either." It looked as if MSKCC's MRI machine might truly have been too sensitive and yielded false positive results.

I was overcome with relief and started to speak, but he cut me off. "Wait," he said, "I have even more good news. The Gleason score on the prostate, when the whole tumor was examined, is now seven, not nine." He was obviously very happy with himself for having done the surgery. He pointed out that a change in the Gleason score after the pathologist had more tissue to examine was common. This changed everything. Now I had a reasonable shot at being cured.

Six weeks later, I went back for my first postoperative PSA. If all the tumor had been removed, there was no prostate tissue to produce PSA, and by six weeks the PSA level should be unmeasurable. This was the next big hurdle for me to clear. If it was measurable, it meant that the surgery hadn't gotten it all, that there was still cancer in my system. We'd have to go on to a new level of treatment. It also meant my chances weren't good. Many more mystery books were consumed in those six weeks.

By the end of the day, Scardino had left me an e-mail. "Vince, I left a message on your cell to let you know that your PSA is undetectable. This is a terrific result and it calls into serious question the significance of the bone lesions seen on the MRI. There is about a 50-50 chance the cancer will not recur for the next 5 years."

Right around the time of my surgery, a big study was published suggesting that postoperative radiotherapy would improve my chances of staying free of disease. We were considering it, but, as often happens to doctors, I got all the postoperative complications you can get. My wound opened and had to be packed daily, I developed deep venous thrombosis and had to go on anti-coagulation medicine, and I went into atrial flutter, a cardiac arrhythmia that required electrical cardioversion to normalize. We shelved the use of postoperative radiotherapy.

But still, I had a shot. Every three months, I went in for a PSA test to see if there was a spike. Every three months, I got the all clear. Until March 15, 2011. On that date, Scardino's e-mail didn't come. I froze, suspecting something was wrong. Sure enough, he called me the next day saying that my recent test had detected a rise in my PSA. He had them repeat it to be sure, hence the delay. He needed to repeat it in a month to see the trend but recommended I now get the postoperative radiotherapy to the tumor bed and the lymph node area as well.

I spent the summer of 2011 in New York City, traveling to Sloan Kettering for radiation five days a week. Ironically, we had built this facility when I was physician in chief of MSKCC. Now I was using it. I commuted to Connecticut on weekends and enjoyed the time off, although I had to laugh at the schedule. I had always teased radiotherapists that treating five days a week was based not on any logic but to ensure them weekends off. Cancer cells grow seven days a week.

I have been fine ever since, though I still have my PSA checked regularly, and it remains undetectable. And, as it does for many people in my position, the worry begins to seep in before each test.

I am lucky, too. I've always said that one of the primary tactics for an oncologist in keeping patients alive is to do so until the next thing comes along. I have leukemic patients alive today because they made it to vincristine and the VAMP program and Hodgkin's patients alive because they made it to MOPP.

When I was diagnosed, hormones were about it for treatment other than radiation and surgery. There was one drug, docetaxel, which had been approved in 2004. When I had my biochemical reoccurrence, we thought about using it. But we decided that given it was the only weapon we had left, we'd hold back and be sure we needed it. As discussed, once a cancer gets habituated to a drug, it can find ways to get around it.

Then there was abiraterone, in 2010, and cabazitaxel, and the first anti-prostate-cancer vaccine, and drugs to inhibit bone metastasis. And then there's enzalutamide, which has an interesting story behind it, with echoes of early days in oncology.

To understand it, let me return to the story of Gleevec, the single-pill therapy used to treat the adult leukemia chronic myeloid leukemia, or CML, previously only treatable in a quarter of cases by bone morrow transplants from matched donors. As you probably remember, it's a targeted therapy, a new-generation drug aimed at a specific genetic error that leads to fusion of the ABL1 gene with an area on another gene, called BCR, which promotes production of an enzyme that causes cells to proliferate into CML.

Most cancers have many genetic errors. CML is unusual in that it's a relatively simple cancer. It does not require as many hits to cause it, and as a result there are fewer targets you have to hit to fix it. Gleevec is a variety of drug known as a kinase inhibitor that blocks the BCR/ABL fusion gene.

It worked almost miraculously at first. But the early patients relapsed. Initially, researchers thought that when patients relapsed, their leukemia was no longer dependent on the BCR gene. What they discovered was that another mutation was occurring that restored the pathway of the original gene's function. This observation led to the development of a second generation of drugs that target the gene.

Charles Sawyers, a physician and scientist at Memorial Sloan Kettering Cancer Center, grew up in the new generation of oncologists, those who knew that there was a molecular basis to cancer. He'd done his Ph.D. with a group of scientists who were hammering out the genetic basis of CML, and he was intimately involved in the development of Gleevec.

After the success of Gleevec, he started wondering about other cancers in which a similar frame of thinking could be applied. Before long, he'd thought of prostate cancer.

Anti-androgen therapy with drugs that block testosterone production has long been a mainstay of treatment for prostate cancer, because testosterone, as I've said, cues cell proliferation, and prostate cancer cells are addicted to it. But the drugs have never been hugely useful, in the long run, because cancer cells appeared to learn to grow without testosterone, entering a stage of disease known as hormone- or androgen-independent prostate cancer.

The thinking was the androgen receptor and drugs that targeted it stopped working because the disease no longer depended on that signaling pathway. But Sawyers thought otherwise. What if the receptors just made do with less hormone?

He developed an animal model to test his hypothesis. Before long, he realized that history was, in fact, repeating itself. It was exactly like what he'd seen with Gleevec. Resistance to hormone therapy was actually due to restored function of androgen receptors. They appeared to be responding to the low levels of androgens still present even while androgens were mostly being blocked with therapy.

To go further was not easy. He had to persuade his lab to study prostate cancer and hormone receptors. Then he had to get the work published, which took eighteen months. Many journals, he says, doubted what he and his lab had found. It was contrary to what most accepted as true about the way that hormone-independent prostate cancer—meaning prostate cancers that had seemingly become immune to testosterone deprivation—worked. And hormones were considered yesterday's drugs.

But he persevered and was successful, largely because of his track record with Gleevec. After that, he began looking into the next generation of inhibitors of the androgen-resistant pathway. First came abiraterone, a drug that reduces androgen levels even further. It was the drug that Lee had missed out on because of tight FDA restrictions. Now there is enzalutamide, the first of a new family of drugs that irreversibly block the androgen receptor itself, preventing androgens from stimulating cell growth. These new drugs, with the promise of more to come, have already revolutionized the treatment of advanced prostate cancer. Suddenly, in a field that had been fallow for decades, there were new options, options that worked better than any that had come before.

That, of course, is the short version. But you get my point. If you aren't hearing echoes of the pessimism that surrounded the development of VAMP and MOPP and Bernie Fisher's difficulty getting his work on lumpectomy versus mastectomy published, you should be.

The bottom line is that I survived because my doctors were courageous in using the tools we already possessed—the oldest tools in the shed, in fact—and that will allow me to take advantage of new ones, should I need them. To my good fortune, where we once had few, we now have many. There are more to come. Hopefully, they will not get too bogged down by our system. The war on cancer is paying off. For me, at seventy-nine, that means my very aggressive prostate cancer, diagnosed more than five years ago, is likely to be, at worst, a chronic disease rather than a fatal one.

There are many more now who could and should be in my position and who are not. Lee was one of them. I wish I had been able to keep him alive a little bit longer, to take advantage of abiraterone. If abiraterone had kept him going longer, he might have made it to enzalutamide and a newer version of the CTLA4 inhibitor, better known as checkpoint inhibitors, now approved for the treatment of melanoma. He was close. Had he had the chance to respond longer with chemotherapy, it might have happened.

All people should get that kind of care. If they did, we'd be curing more. We can cure more. And we will win the war on cancer. The death of cancer is inevitable. It is a question not of if but of when. And when will be determined by what we do next. Do it now or do it later. Many are resigned to later.

Recently, at a dinner for the FDA commissioner, I sat next to an outstanding clinical investigator who works with the exciting new drugs recently available for advanced melanoma. For the first time in my long career, we are seeing remissions that are likely cures of this ferocious disease. I asked my dinner companion how he was affected by all the regulations that have been piled on by the FDA and the NCI. He said, "Vince, if they would leave me alone, I could cure so many more patients."

I was startled. "Really?" I said. "Really," he answered.

Then he waved his hand, as if dismissing the conversation. "But it'll happen in five years, anyway."

We have become resigned, those of us who treat cancer, to the delays. But should we be? Certainly patients fighting for their lives, who need these new therapies now, do not feel this way. They don't have time for it.

The rate-limiting step in eradicating cancer today is not the science but the regulatory environment we work in.

I confess, I am not resigned to later.

In 1971, when the National Cancer Act was passed, we had not yet arrived at critical mass, as Mary Lasker thought we had. It was one of her rare miscalculations. But it was as good a time as any to launch a concerted effort to conquer this disease, and the money provided by the war on cancer got us here—to real critical mass—much, much faster than we would otherwise have done. The truth is, the war on cancer has been one of the most successful government programs ever. But we have outgrown the original act, and we need a new one, with a new organization. It can and should be done.

At the least, a new act should call for the creation of a new position, a cancer czar, with budget authority over all government components of the cancer program and an office in the Executive Office Building adjacent to the White House. The original cancer act called the war on cancer the National Cancer Program. I was appointed director of the National Cancer Program in addition to director of the NCI. The framers did this because they envisioned the program expanding beyond the confines of the NCI. And they were correct. Not only is there today a very significant component in private industry, but hundreds of millions of dollars of support for cancer research now exists in the Defense Department, the Centers for Disease Control, and other agencies. There is no coordination among the different entities. One hand doesn't know what the other is doing. A czar would finally allow the cancer program to set and manage its own priorities.

The NCI's Cancer Centers Program should be able to operate the way it was originally designed to. There were only three cancer centers when the act was passed, so the framers had to look into the future. Here is what they envisioned: an expanded network of cancer centers that would have sufficient geographic distribution so that every cancer patient could reach a cancer center if he or she needed special care.

And a comprehensive center would be just that—an institution that is research oriented but that could bring the full panoply of research to the bedside. A freestanding, independent entity.

The centers are tightly overregulated by both the NCI and the FDA. Combination anti-hallmark therapy? Forget it.

The FDA and the NCI should delegate all authority for early clinical trials (phases I and II) to cancer centers. Modern approaches to developing clinical trials require flexibility and the ability to adjust protocols on the run. Each center deserves the right to have the equivalent of its own Society of Jabbering Idiots. Most important is the fact that far more expertise exists at cancer centers than at the NCI and the FDA combined. Today we have the tail wagging the dog. And as a result, we are depriving cancer patients of what they—and their families—want most. A chance. We are losing too many people who should not be lost.

Finally, the method of funding centers needs to be reexamined. The current mechanism is archaic. It was set up forty years ago and hasn't changed since. Cancer center directors should have real authority over all NCI-funded programs at their institutions to allow them to build truly functional research programs.

What I have been describing for you in this book is not news to many on the inside of this war. In fact, much of what I've been describing for you here is an open secret among doctors and administrators who prefer not to air it to the public, because they either don't want you to know, or think you couldn't possibly be interested, or think it's too complicated, or are afraid it will negatively impact their careers.

But that has, in my opinion, merely resulted in confusion, at best, and, at worst, the whiplashing of the American public as they read about both advances in the war on cancer and the "failed war on cancer." The truth is much more complex and much more hopeful.

In 1998, I met with John Seffrin, the CEO of the American Cancer Society, and his deputy, a former trainee of mine, Dr. Harmon Eyre, to discuss the creation of a new organization to try to save the war on cancer. The plan was to ask former president George H. W. Bush, who had lost a daughter to cancer, to serve as chair of a new organization called the National Dialogue on Cancer, whose purpose would be to get all the major advocacy groups to speak with one voice to reactivate the cancer act. He agreed and, to make it a bipartisan effort, asked Senator Dianne Feinstein to act as co-chair.

After an initial planning session, a meeting of about one hundred people representing every group with an interest in cancer was held in 1999 in Washington, D.C. The then-director of the NCI, Rick Klausner, who sat next to me, spent most of the morning talking in my ear sotto voce about what a waste of time the meeting was.

Senator Feinstein asked me to co-chair a new committee with John Seffrin, commissioned by the senator to rewrite the cancer act for the new millennium.

The deliberations were dominated by the advocacy groups, and most of the debate focused on protecting the interests of existing organizations. In the end, the committee recommended a new, expanded organizational structure to coordinate the country's efforts in the war on cancer, although the resistance to this, especially from the NCI, which would have lost its primacy in the new organization, was fierce.

The completed proposal was presented to the current president, George W. Bush, in the week of September 10, 2001. A day later, terrorists flew planes into the World Trade Center and the Pentagon, and the president and the rest of the country got distracted by another war. Later, a committee of the Senate, chaired by Senator Ted Kennedy, reexamined the passage of a new cancer act. Again, advocacy groups protecting their own interests dominated the process. The last draft that I saw looked like a laundry list of tired old programs.

Despite this, the war on cancer forges ahead—albeit in more cumbersome fashion than it should. And I still get e-mails and phone calls from patients who have found my name on the Internet or an academic paper or seen me quoted somewhere, asking for help. Often I can, but just as often I am frustrated by obstacles that I know should not be there.

And still, in the midst of these calls for help, I receive e-mails, letters, and phone calls from the people who took part in the original MOPP study. At first, these letters were about their survival and then, often, their marriages and the births of their children and, years later, their grandchildren. Though I have kept all their letters, I have not seen most of my former patients since they came to the NIH as teenagers and young adults.

Whenever I receive a new letter or e-mail, two things cross my mind. The first is that in any war there are a handful of heroes, people who risked everything for the cause. There are a handful of doctors in this category, people like Jay Freireich and Bernie Fisher, who risked everything to save people. They have endured and finally received the acclaim that was always their due. But it is the patients who were the real heroes of the early war on cancer. They often thank me, but really we should all be thanking them.

The second thing I think is something I rarely put into words. How can I tell these people, who reach out to share their lives, that while I remember them clearly and cherish their missives, it is the ones who are not here whose memory I carry with me most vividly?

NOTES

1. Outrageous Fortune

1. Alexandre R. Zlotta et al., "Prevalence of Prostate Cancer on Autopsy: Cross-Sectional Study on Unscreened Caucasian and Asian Men," *Journal of the National Cancer Institute*, published online July 11, 2013, http://jnci.oxfordjournals.org/content/early/2013/07/05/jnci.djt151.full.pdf+html.

2. H. Zincke et al., "Long-Term (15 Years) Results After Radical Prostatectomy for Clinically Localized (Stage T2c or Lower) Prostate Cancer," *Journal of Urology* 152, no. 5 (1994): 1850–57.

3. James G. Herman et al., "Silencing of the VHL Tumor-Suppressor Gene by DNA Methylation in Renal Carcinoma," *Proceedings of the National Academy of Sciences of the United States of America* 91, no. 21 (1994): 9700–9704.

4. Gerhardt Attard et al., "Phase I Clinical Trial of a Selective Inhibitor of CYP17, Abiraterone Acetate, Confirms That Castration-Resistant Prostate Cancer Commonly Remains Hormone Driven," *Journal of Clinical Oncology* 26, no. 28 (2008): 4563–71.

5. Howard Scher et al., "Adaptive Clinical Trial Designs for Simultaneous Testing of Matched Diagnostics and Therapeutics," *Clinical Cancer Research* 17, no. 21 (2011): 6634–40.

2. The Chemotherapists

1. Alfred Gellhorn and Erich Hirschberg, eds., "Investigation of Diverse Systems of Cancer Chemotherapy Screening," *Cancer Research Supplement* 3 (1955).

2. Kenneth Endicott, "Progress Report, Bethesda (MD): Cancer Chemotherapy," *National Service Center* (1957): 10; Kenneth Endicott, "The Chemotherapy Program," *Journal of*

the National Cancer Institute 19 (1957): 275–93; C. Gordon Zubrod et al., "The Chemotherapy Program of the National Cancer Institute: History, Analysis, and Plans," *Cancer Chemotherapy Reports* 50 (1966): 349–540.

3. Sidney Farber et al., "Temporary Remissions in Acute Leukemia in Children Produced by Folic Acid Antagonist, 4-Aminopteroyl-Glutamic Acid (Aminopterin)," *New England Journal of Medicine* 238 (1948): 787–93.

4. O. H. Pearson et al., "ACTH- and Cortisone-Induced Regression of Lymphoid Tumors in Man: A Preliminary Report," *Cancer* 2, no. 6 (1949): 943–45.

5. George H. Hitchings and Gertrude B. Elion, "The Chemistry and Biochemistry of Purine Analogs," *Annals of the New York Academy of Sciences* 60 (1954): 195–99.

6. Howard Skipper et al., "Implications of Biochemical, Cytokinetic, Pharmacologic, and Toxicologic Relationships in the Design of Optimal Therapeutic Schedules," *Cancer Chemotherapy Reports* 54 (1950): 431–50.

3. MOMP

1. Emil Freireich et al., "Quadruple Combination Therapy (VAMP) for Acute Lymphocytic Leukemia of Childhood," *Proceedings of the American Association for Cancer Research* 5 (1964): 20.

2. Phillip Frost and Vincent DeVita, "Pigmentation due to a New Antitumor Agent: Effects of Topical Application of BCNU (1,3-Bis [2-Chloroethyl]-1-Nitrosourea)," *Archives of Dermatology* 94, no. 3 (1966): 265–68.

3. Thomas Hodgkin, "On Some Morbid Appearances of the Absorbent Glands and Spleen," *Medico-chirurgical Transactions* 17 (1832): 69–97.

4. D. M. Reed, "On the Pathological Changes in Hodgkin's Disease, with Especial Reference to Its Relation to Tuberculosis," *Johns Hopkins Hospital Reports* 10 (1902): 133–96.

5. Eric C. Easson and Marion H. Russell, "The Cure of Hodgkin's Disease," *British Medical Journal* 1 (1963): 1704–7.

6. *Trials of War Criminals Before the Nuremberg Military Tribunals Under Control Council Law No. 10* (Washington, D.C.: U.S. Government Printing Office, 1949), 2:181–82.

4. MOPP

1. Vincent DeVita and Arthur Serpick, "Combination Chemotherapy in the Treatment of Advanced Hodgkin's Disease," abstract 49, *Proceedings of the American Association for Cancer Research* 8 (1967): 13.

2. Vincent DeVita et al., "Combination Chemotherapy of Advanced Hodgkin's Disease: The NCI Program—a Progress Report," abstract 73, *Proceedings of the American Association for Cancer Research* 10 (1969): 19.

3. Ibid.

4. Vincent DeVita et al., "Combination Chemotherapy in the Treatment of Advanced Hodgkin's Disease," *Annals of Internal Medicine* 73, no. 6 (1970): 881–95.

5. Walt Kelly, *Pogo: We Have Met the Enemy and He Is Us* (New York: Simon & Schuster, 1972).

5. The War on Cancer

1. National Cancer Act of 1971, National Cancer Institute, dtp.nci.nih.gov/timeline /noflash/milestones/m4_nixon.htm.

6. Boots on the Ground

1. George P. Canellos et al., "Cyclical Combination Chemotherapy in the Treatment of Advanced Breast Carcinoma," *British Medical Journal* 1 (1974): 218–20.

2. Bernard Fisher et al., "L-Phenylalanine Mustard (L-PAM) in the Management of Primary Breast Cancer—a Report of Early Findings," *New England Journal of Medicine* 292 (1975): 117–22.

3. Vincent DeVita et al., "Advanced Diffuse Histiocytic Lymphoma, a Potentially Curable Disease: Results with Combination Chemotherapy," *Lancet* 1, no. 7901 (1975): 248–50.

4. James D. Watson, "To Fight Cancer, Know the Enemy," *New York Times*, August 6, 2009, A29.

5. Nils J. Bruzelius, "U.S. Cancer Program Termed 'Sham,'" *Boston Globe*, March 7, 1975, 1.

6. Editorial, "Dissent Against the War on Cancer," *Baltimore Sun*, April 16, 1975, A16.

7. Harold M. Schmeck Jr., "War on Cancer Stirs a Political Backlash," *The New York Times*, May 27, 1975.

8. Nicholas von Hoffman, "False Front in War on Cancer," *Chicago Tribune*, February 13, 1975, A3.

7. Cleaning House at the National Cancer Institute

1. Jonathan Neumann and Ted Gup, "Experimental Drugs: Death in the Search for Cures," *The Washington Post*, October 18, 1981, 1; Jonathan Neumann and Ted Gup, "Risk, Rivalry and Research—and Error," *Washington Post*, October 19, 1981, A1; Jonathan Neumann and Ted Gup, "The World of Shattered Hopes," *The Washington Post*, October 20, 1981, 1.

2. S. Kister et al., "An Analysis of Predictor Variables for Adjuvant Treatment of Breast Cancer," *Cancer Chemotherapy and Pharmacology* 2, no. 3 (1979): 147–58, www.rand.org/pubs/external_publications/EP19790001.html.

3. Peter Greenwald and Edward Sondik, eds., *Cancer Control Objectives for the Nation: 1985–2000*, National Cancer Institute Monographs 2 (Bethesda, Md.: National Cancer Institute, 1986).

8. Frances Kelsey Syndrome

1. Frances Oldham Kelsey, Chemical Heritage Foundation, www.chemheritage.org/discover/online-resources/chemistry-in-history/themes/public-and-environmental-health/food-and-drug-safety/kelsey.aspx.

2. Morton Mintz, "'Heroine' of FDA Keeps Bad Drug off Market," *Washington Post*, July 15, 1962.

3. Attard et al., "Phase I Clinical Trial of a Selective Inhibitor of CYP17, Abiraterone Acetate, Confirms That Castration-Resistant Prostate Cancer Commonly Remains Hormone Driven."

4. Abigail Alliance for Better Access to Developmental Drugs v. Eschenbach, www.wlf.org/litigating/case_detail.asp?id=266.

5. U.S. Food and Drug Administration Oncologic Drugs Advisory Committee, www.fda.gov/AdvisoryCommittees/CommitteesMeetingMaterials/Drugs/Oncologic DrugsAdvisoryCommittee.

6. *Cancer Letter*, April 27, 2007. The ODAC meeting took place on March 29, 2007.

7. Gustave Le Bon, *The Crowd: A Study of the Popular Mind* (London: T. Fisher Unwin, 1896; originally published as *La psychologie des foules* [Paris: F. Alcan, 1895]).

8. David M. Dilts and Alan B. Sandler, "Invisible Barriers to Clinical Trials: The Impact of Structural, Infrastructural, and Procedural Barriers to Opening Oncology Clinical Trials," *Journal of Clinical Oncology* 24, no. 28 (2006): 4545–52.

9. "The U.S. Food and Drug Administration today approved Zytiga (abiraterone acetate) in combination with prednisone (a steroid) to treat patients with late-stage (metastatic) castration-resistant prostate cancer who have received prior docetaxel (chemotherapy)." PRNewswire-USNewswire, news release, April 28, 2011.

10. The Death of Cancer

1. Sharon Begley, "Rethinking the War on Cancer," *Newsweek*, September 5, 2008, www.newsweek.com/rethinking-war-cancer-88941.

2. Gina Kolata, "Forty Years' War: Advances Elusive in the Drive to Cure Cancer," *New York Times*, April 23, 2009, www.nytimes.com/2009/04/24/health/policy/24cancer.html?_r=0.

3. Clifton Leaf, *The Truth in Small Doses: Why We're Losing the War on Cancer—and How to Win It* (New York: Simon & Schuster, 2013).

4. Kevin M. Murphy and Robert H. Topel, "The Value of Health and Longevity," *Journal of Political Economy* 114, no. 5 (2006): 871.

5. Douglas Hanahan and Robert A. Weinberg, "Hallmarks of Cancer: The Next Generation," *Cell* 144, no. 5 (2011): 646–74.

6. Robert A. Weinberg, *The Biology of Cancer*, vol. 1 (New York: Garland Science, 2007).

7. Douglas Hanahan and Robert A. Weinberg, "The Hallmarks of Cancer," *Cell* 100, no. 1 (2000): 57–70.

8. Jacob P. Laubach et al., "The Evolution and Impact of Therapy in Multiple Myeloma," supplement, *Medical Oncology* 27, no. S1 (2010): S1–S6.

9. Shyamala Maheswaran et al., "Detection of Mutations in *EGFR* in Circulating Lung-Cancer Cells," *New England Journal of Medicine* 359 (2008): 366–77.

10. David Z. Chang et al., "Phase I Trial of Capecitabine in Combination with Interferon Alpha in Patients with Metastatic Renal Cancer: Toxicity and Pharmacokinetics," *Cancer Chemotherapy and Pharmacology* 48, no. 6 (2001): 493–98.

11. G. H. J. Mickisch et al., "Radical Nephrectomy plus Interferon-Alfa-Based Immunotherapy Compared with Interferon Alfa Alone in Metastatic Renal-Cell Carcinoma: A Randomised Trial," *Lancet* 358, no. 9286 (2001): 966–70.

12. Weill Cornell Newsroom, "Keeping Cancer from Fertile Ground: Weill Cornell Team Identifies Key Players in 'Pre-metastasis'; Groundbreaking Work Could Lead to New Drug Targets and Methods of Assessing Cancer Recurrence Risk," press release, December 7, 2005.

13. Dana R. Leach et al., "Enhancement of Antitumor Immunity by CTLA-4 Blockade," *Science* 271, no. 5256 (1996): 1734–36.

14. Eric Tran et al., "Cancer Immunotherapy Based on Mutation-Specific CD4+ T Cells in a Patient with Epithelial Cancer," *Science* 344, no. 6184 (2014): 641–45.

15. James N. Kochenderfer et al., "B-Cell Depletion and Remissions of Malignancy along with Cytokine-Associated Toxicity in a Clinical Trial of Anti-CD19 Chimeric-Antigen-Receptor-Transduced T cells," *Blood* 119, no. 12 (2012): 2709–20.

Writing a memoir is an opportunity to look back and acknowledge people who had a positive impact on your life and career. In my case, I'd have to start with my mother, Isabella DeVita, who, by the time I was seven, was determined that I should become a doctor, and my father, who always proudly supported me. Medicine turned out to be a good fit for me, although I think my mother envisioned me carrying a black bag and making house calls. I am nonetheless grateful to them, always.

Despite her determination, medical school wouldn't have happened without the help of a few key figures in my history. In high school I took a trip on the wild side, for a time, until Henry (Hank) Richards, the very effective and lovable principal of Roosevelt High School in Yonkers, New York, took me aside and, in one short meeting, set me back on a path to college. The same thing happened in my sophomore year at the College of William and Mary. My path to medical school was salvaged by a very determined professor of chemistry, Alfred Armstrong, who cornered me on campus one day and confronted me about my flagging grades. His tough chemistry courses ultimately made lab courses in medical school easy for me.

At the George Washington School of Medicine, C. Adrian Hogben, the newly appointed chairman of Physiology, saw something in me I didn't see myself, and gave me my first opportunity to do lab research at Mt. Desert Island Biological Laboratory in Bar Harbor, Maine. There, Hogben introduced me to Dave Rall, who took me into the fold at the National Cancer Institute. During my training in internal medicine at Yale, the great Paul Beeson gave me the confidence to question dogma and believe in what I saw more than in what I was told.

But the biggest impact on my career came from two men who were no strangers to the wild side themselves—the pioneering oncologists Tom Frei and Jay Freireich, most especially Jay, who served as a role model of a caring yet aggressive cancer doctor and researcher. Jay and Tom, the Bobbsey Twins, as my colleague and friend George Canellos, nicknamer extraordinaire, dubbed them, laid the groundwork for Jack Moxley and me to think big and out of the box when beginning our work with combination chemotherapy of Hodgkin's disease. I have fond memories of working with Jack in those early days.

Working with my colleagues in the Medicine Branch—George Canellos, Bruce Chabner, Phil Schein, and Bob Young ("the gang of five," as we euphemistically called ourselves) when I was Chief of Medicine at NCI was a not-to-be-forgotten and exhilarating experience. I'm grateful to all of them. I am also indebted to my friend and colleague Steve Rosenberg, Chief of Surgery at NCI, for all his support, not to mention his medical advice, and for constantly prodding me to write this book.

Working with my daughter Elizabeth has been one of the most rewarding experiences of my career. The extent to which the stories here depict real life I owe to Elizabeth's extraordinary writing skills. She taught me a lot about writing.

And without the encouragement and support of my loving wife, Mary Kay DeVita, who patiently listened to and commented on the same stories as we refined them, the book and much of the good that I have been blessed with would not have happened. I am also grateful to my friends Amy and Joe Perella for endowing my chair at Yale, giving me the flexibility to write this book.

I owe special thanks to our dear friend Barbara, who allowed us to share Lee's story (and hers). And to my assistant, Andrea Perrelli, who labored long hours over the manuscript, and to Zia Raven, whose searching skills are unsurpassed. I would also like to thank Paul Raeburn, whose sage advice on every aspect of the preparation of the book was invaluable. Also, our thanks to Mindy Werner for her very helpful editorial insight; and to the Invisible Institute for its infinite support to Elizabeth.

And finally, the wise counsel of both Sarah Crichton, our editor, and her assistant, Marsha Sasmor, as well as that of Mark Reiter, our agent, every step of the way, from design to publication, has been greatly appreciated.

Vincent DeVita
New Haven, Connecticut